# Living In a Brainstorm

Erica Egge

Living In a Brainstorm

A memoir

First edition, July 2013
Moos Girls Publishing House

ISBN: 978-0-9895380-1-5

# Prologue

## Storytelling

Storytelling is an important part of the human experience. We use stories to pass down the wisdom learned throughout history. We tell stories of joy, stories of hardship, stories of triumph, stories of failure. We listen to stories to help us, to guide us; we tell stories to help us, to purge us. I'm telling a story. I'm telling a story of me, of my life. I want to tell the world, or anyone who feels like listening, about my thoughts, dreams, fears, happiness, and my pursuit of courage. Telling my story might help someone else, and if that comes true, every breath I take as I type these words is precious to me. But even if the great blue yonder of the blogosphere echoes only to me, telling my story helps bring me peace. Hello, my name is Erica, and I am an epileptic. I have seizures, and they have shaped my life. I have seizures, and they have made me who I am. I take fifteen pills a day, and they give me debilitating side effects. I take fifteen pills a day, and I still have seizures. My name is Erica, I am an epileptic, I have seizures, I take fifteen pills a day, it has shaped who I am, but it is not who I am. I live a full and happy life. I ate food off the floor as a kid and built up a great immune system, so I rarely get sick. I am blessed with amazing friends and an amazing family. I live a full and happy life. My name is Erica, I have debilitating side effects, I still have seizures, and I am doing something about it. I am going to have two scary, hard surgeries, and I am telling my story. Maybe I'll touch someone, maybe I won't, but I'll try. Either way, bearing myself, unfiltered and exposed, telling my story raw, makes me see myself for who I am and how I feel. Telling my story gives me strength.

My name is Erica, and this is my story.

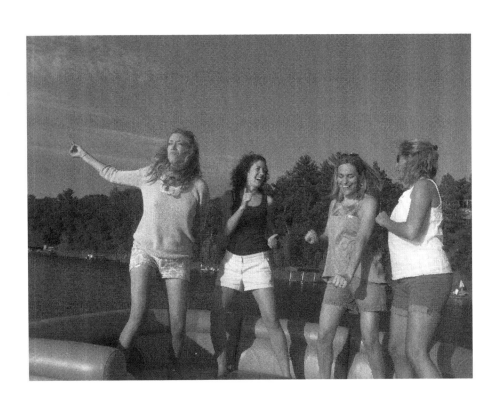

# Part I: Decisions

For my sisters and my friends for their support, smiles, strength and kindness.

October, 2010

## It Started With a Dress

Like most great things do. Grey with white piping, it hung unused in the dress section of my closet. I had left my job unexpectedly less than a week before. I'd shown up one day, realized how unhappy I was, not to mention I hated selling phones, and something told me to run. So I quit. I hadn't planned to as I carefully dried my hair and applied my makeup that morning, but when I got there, I knew that that was not where I was supposed to be anymore. The only problem was that I never got to wear my gray dress.

I held up the hanger and contemplated the dress, abandoned and obsolete with the price tag still hanging from its beautiful seam. Throwing caution to the wind, I cut the plastic string that held the paper to it, and contorted my arms to zip it up my back. Dress codes be damned, I added a belt and boots and went to Starbucks.

Over the past couple months, I'd been having severe side effects from my seizure meds that had affected my job quite noticeably. Dizziness, double vision, nausea and fatigue followed me around as I held on to the wall to steady myself to walk from my desk to the break room; walking around the office in a zig-zag pattern at 9am is frustrating and embarrassing. During the day, I occasionally had to park my car in an Arby's parking lot and nap, leaning my head against the steering wheel and trying not to wrinkle my suit, because I was literally unable to keep my eyes open. In meetings, I would have to pause and pretend I dropped my pen to hide the seizure I was having. Never in my life had I been so acutely aware of my epilepsy. I thought about that as I sat with my venti skim toffee latte (my favorite barista there always concocted drinks for me with too many adjectives that I stopped paying attention and just enjoyed it). My computer sat on the small table in front of me, urging me to re-open my JobFinder account and find another job. Stop wasting time, Erica. Stop wasting your life, Erica. Be productive, Erica. Hurry up, Erica! I spent two hours looking at jobs in law enforcement and finance, but then my fingers began to itch; there was something I was overlooking. Tentatively, looking around like a kid reading a comic inside a geometry book, I opened a new tab and searched "epilepsy surgery". It was a rush like none other when the page filled up with descriptions, forums, diagrams and hospitals. I dug deeper, clicking on the first link, and thought, can I do this? I kind of think I want to...

An hour later I'd fallen through the rabbit hole; I was hooked. A new patron walked through the door, throwing a gust of cold October air that rustled the ink-covered pages of my notebook, and I made my decision. I was going to have brain surgery.


## Memories

I remember my first seizure clearly. My little sister, Greta, and I were sitting at a little white plastic table in our bedroom at the cabin, drawing pictures in colors from Crayola's big crayon box, which spans the entirety of the light spectrum. Suddenly, my right arm got a funny feeling in it and began to move on it's own. It started on the table and swept side to side, pushing all of the crayons and sheets of recycled paper onto the floor. It continued for about fifteen seconds, then stopped. We looked at it, stunned, and after a beat Greta bounced up and down, smiling and saying, "do it again, Erica!" I looked at my arm, swatted it with my other hand, and said, "do it again, arm! Do it again!" My arm didn't oblige that day, but it would another. We picked up our drawings and the crayons, which had rolled down the uneven floor to rest under the radiator, and continued our activity until it was time for dinner. I remember thinking it was funny while it happened and while it amused my sister, but as the hands on the clock moved, the sun began to set, and the house smelled of green beans, grilled chicken and mac and cheese, my amusement turned to curiosity, to confusion, to anxiety, to fear. What happened to me? I knew that it wasn't right, but I had no idea what it was. And I was scared. Over the next year, until I was diagnosed, and even a while after, I cried every time I had a seizure. For a six year old, going from hospital to hospital but still not knowing why my arm was shaking was terrifying. I was terrified.

I don't say this to get sympathy. The object of telling this is simply to begin my story. Living with undiagnosed epilepsy is a scary thing, so when you finally do learn what's happening, it's relieving. From that day on, epilepsy becomes a part of who you are. It shapes you and your outlook on life in a way you couldn't have imagined. You're more aware of your body and your schedule. You're cognizant of your diet and your lifestyle. But mostly, you're much more aware and sensitive to other people with disabilities. Comments about retards and diabetes and AIDS suddenly aren't that funny. Jokes about someone's dancing making them look like they're having a seizure don't make you laugh. It might even make you nauseous.

The unknown is composed of anxiety and trust. Yesterday, I scheduled an appointment for a consultation and extensive testing to find where exactly my seizures originate so that it can be taken out while I lie asleep on a table. I don't know how long I'll be there. I don't know if I'll have the surgery during that visit or if I'll be coming back a week later. Two weeks later. I don't know how long the recovery will be or what it's going to entail. I don't know how long I should plan on subletting my apartment in Denver while I stay with my parents in Minnesota, an hour and a half away from The Mayo Clinic. Or maybe it'll turn out that I'm not a candidate for surgery. That would break my heart. My unknown future is filled with unsolvable variables that make me anxious beyond belief, but it's full to the brim with trust. Trust that this surgery will be worth every ounce of worry and then some. It's still scary, but every part of my future that is given a diagnosis is a relief.


## It's All About Me

Sometimes I forget that it's not all about me. My life impacts so many other lives, just the way theirs impact mine. When one of my best friends told me she got engaged, I almost fell off my chair in excitement. And when that same friend's mom spent a week in the hospital, I was so worried I lost my appetite. As much as I take those reactions - happiness, sadness, excitement, anxiety, pride - for granted, it doesn't register in my mind that others feel the same protectiveness of me. Why should they? I'm not a wife, certainly not a mom, not an employee, not a roommate, not a therapist, so where do I fit? No one is financially dependent on me, no one is counting on me to raise them, or shrink them. I rely so heavily on the love and support of my friends and family precisely because I don't fit anywhere yet, and I would do anything to keep them safe. When your situation in life doesn't make you responsible for anyone, you adopt. I have adopted my friends and my family as cubs to my mama bear. So then why do they treat me like a cub? Why would my safety and happiness be such a strong concern of theirs? Because that's just how it works, silly rabbit. Love isn't about trying to fit in. Love transcends the boxes you checked on the Census mail out. Chances are that when you care deeply about someone, they care about you, too. When your heart is full of people you love, it's hard to imagine that that many people could love you back. But guess what? They do. Not one person on this earth could really know how many people their life affects. How many people depend on them existing, growing, thriving. Living.

Yesterday over a bowl of cereal and a foot-long To Do list, my sister gave me one of those, "are you stupid or something?" looks that only a big sister can give. Since announcing that I'm having brain surgery, my friends and family have said that they're nervous, but they think I've made the right choice and support me. It wasn't until today, though, that I actually got that. My sister Coco and I were talking about leasing my apartment in Denver to go live with our parents in Minnesota for my surgery and through the recovery, but when I said I'd sublet it for December and January, she stopped, spoon half raised, and asked out loud, "What's wrong with you?" Thanks, sis. "Why do you think you could go back to Denver after January?", pause, are you stupid or something look. She reminded me that my recovery isn't going to take four weeks. I definitely won't be in any shape to live alone by then. Though I hate being wrong, I admitted she was right. "I don't want to live at home for a whole month before it though," I whined. I knew it would be best since I'd be nearby in case I had to go to any extra doctor appointments or do any testing on short notice, but still. Live with my parents? As much as we're very close and as much as I love them, all I could think about was getting nagged. "Coco, dad's just gonna spend all the time asking me about my job search and what I'm gonna do with my life." But then a funny thing happened. "No, he's not," she said, completely seriously and with full conviction. I didn't realize before how right she must be. For once, my dad doesn't care about my job. He's scared. Both of my parents are scared. My sisters are scared. The rest of my family is scared. My friends are scared. They're scared because once I'm wheeled into the OR, there's nothing more they can do. They'll be totally helpless. All over the country, they'll pace and they'll pray. I never realized how much I matter, how much I really do matter, until I began to see all of the brave faces around me, hanging on to faith, hope, each other, to keep on the smile that gives me the confidence to go through with this. I was so thankful for all of them. I finally started to get it, and I loved them back with all my heart.

As I sat in Coco's kitchen with my bowl of cereal, I realized something about those brave faces. I thought about my decision to have surgery, and started to understand one of the reasons they were scared - they were surprised. I told them that I was going to have surgery for my epilepsy. I didn't ask their advice, or even warn them that I'd been thinking about it, I just sprang it on them - a declaration from a stubborn mouth about her stubborn brain. I realized then that they deserved an explanation, some clarification, proof that I'd thought this over, that it wasn't just a whim. I have a tendency to get flustered on the phone when I try to explain something. I get defensive easily and quickly. Therefore, I decided to give my explanation to my family in an email. I know how impersonal that sounds, but I knew that that was my best chance to let them into my head and get them to understand why I was doing what I was about to do.

## Impulsive

Dear family,

The realization/transformation in my life that made me quit my job and decide to have brain surgery has come at the same time that I've noticed more and more the things that I can't do because of my epilepsy. In the past I was fine with it, I accepted that I have limitations that other people don't, but lately it's become a flashing red stop sign in front of so many things I want to do. It stares me down everyday, and I'm over it. I'm done. I take fifteen pills a day, some of which give me side effects to the point where I can't stand up and walk straight for hours. I'll be incapacitated for almost a whole day, and when I get to the point where I'm feeling okay, it's time to take my next dose. I feel like Sisyphus with a boulder of seizures and anticonvulsants. I've been a perfect candidate for surgery for more than ten years, but I've never felt the need until now. The most frustrating feeling is not being able to finish a sentence because I forget what I said, or what I was going to say, or the word I'm trying to use. I feel like I'm mediocre at everything I do because I know I can do something better but I can't remember how. The reason I get so frustrated when trying to make a point to you is that I feel like you're telling me to do something I've already done or already plan to, but I'm now realizing that maybe I'm not able to convey at the start what I've done and what I plan to do. I'm not able to make the point in my head come out in a comprehensive manner. I'm trapped inside my mind, and I just can't do it anymore. I've gone through Lord knows how many medications. I'm on so many of them right now, but I'm still having seizures. Every day. I can't do this anymore. Something needs to change. With surgery, there's a minimum 70% chance that I'll never have another seizure and won't have to take medicine anymore. I can't even imagine that; it would be a whole new life. A whole new world. That is why I suddenly have said that I'm going to have surgery. It's not all of a sudden, it's so many things that have always been there but have finally become too much for me to handle.

I've often heard that your 20's is the hardest age in life. Despite being agile and having great skin, in your 20's you have no idea what you're doing. It's like being in middle school again. You're still trying to figure out who you are and what's important to you. I'm there now, searching for my place in the world. I've come to realize that my happiness is one of the most important parts of that. I know some of the decisions I make seem unexpected and impulsive, but I promise, they are well thought out. I know what I'm doing. I know what parts I don't know and have plans for how I can learn about them. It all happens in my head behind my ability to verbalize, which makes it difficult for me to explain it to you. I'm hoping this email and the blog I'm starting will allow me to set my ideas and my plans out in a way that you can see and understand them. Hopefully this has shed light onto some things and makes you feel more comfortable with me.

I love you,

Erica


## Coming Into Focus

You'd think that 25 years in, I would accept when something abstract turns into something real. I would understand that that's how the world works. That's what happens every time that we carry out a decision. Decide to try a new recipe for dinner and then follow through. Decide to move your arm and suddenly it lifts up from your lap. These daily transformations of thought to action, contemplation to actualization, don't surprise me. I understand them. But somehow there still exist ideas that catch me off guard when all of a sudden they become real. An abstract cloud in my mind turns to conversation, but once it becomes real, it catches me off guard. My romantic notions disappear as it comes into focus and I see all of the bold lines and sharp edges. Today I scheduled the first step toward a brain surgery. My vision of the conclusion, no more seizures, has expanded to show all of the steps that will come before that glorious new life can start. It's becoming real. On December 23rd, 2010, I'll be going to The Mayo Clinic in Rochester, Minnesota, for a couple days of testing and a consultation with a neurologist. The 23rd is a Friday this year. I'll be packing a bag with my clothes, my toothbrush, and hopefully a little plastic tree to remind me that it will be Christmas soon. My spirits sank when I realized that I won't be wearing a Santa hat and handing out presents from beneath a huge Christmas tree, decorated with ornaments that we made at a church gathering in third grade. I won't be having my mom's beef stroganoff with shoe string potatoes. Instead, I'll be in a hospital bed, thinking about the tests to come and the drill and knives that will follow them. But then I remembered, I'll be vulnerable, scared and needing help just in time for Jesus to come. Pretty good timing, no? I'll have someone in my corner, holding my hand as I go through the process. Being in the hospital just in time for Christmas isn't about missing beef or Santa hats or brightly wrapped boxes covered in pine needles. No, being in the hospital for Christmas will make me stop and remember what Christmas is really about. I'll be like the Whos down in Whoville.

I keep pausing and looking at December 23rd in my calendar. "Seven forty five am - Mayo." Wendy, the neurology department scheduling assistant, said that I should expect to be in the hospital for three to seven business days. The first day will be a consultation, which will determine how long I'll be lying in bed wearing polka dotted hospital gowns and catching up on seasons 1-12 of Law and Order: SVU. After that, I'll go through a series of tests to complete my brain mapping so they know exactly where my seizures originate and can take it out. Then I'll likely have the surgery, and then stay in the hospital for a little while to make sure I'm alright and everything went according to plan. Once I'm cleared to leave, I'll go back to my parents' house to recover. I'll be catatonic for a week or so, then just healing for a few weeks. Maybe a couple months. Finally, after all of the sharp edges that have so boldly come into focus, I'll be free. I'll have a new life. I still can't imagine what it will be like. Though I waver as I stand, and my feet become nervous and unsteady, I have to remember the reason I'm doing this. I have to remember that the bold lines and sharp edges are only part of the picture. The bright future still shines through.


**Whirlwind**


Ok. It's ok, Erica. Breathe. I talked to the scheduling assistant at Mayo's neuro department, and she told me that the doctor can get me in on November 24th. The appointment is at 12:30, but I'll need to be there at 11:45 to register. Ok. Wow. That's great, right? Of course that's great, it's almost exactly a month earlier than originally planned. This way I can get this over with and move on even sooner. So why is my brow furrowed and my mind spinning? This is good. Erica, calm down. This is what you wanted, right? Of course it's what I want. And I really do want it and I really am happy, I'm just overwhelmed. There's so much to do before then, and now I only have four weeks in which to get everything figured out.

The appointment is for the consultation with the doctor, the testing, and the monitoring. The surgery, assuming I'm approved, won't be in that visit. I asked if she could guess when it would be, if it was closer to a week later or more like a couple months later. She said she wishes she could tell me, but it depends on what the doctor says. It depends. Everything depends. Can't I find out anything? My to do list spans out in front of me, like one of those scrolls in a cartoon that rolls out farther and farther and farther to reveal the longest, most daunting amount of information you've ever seen. So far, the list I've assembled in the past few hours includes: find someone to sublet my place in Denver; pack all of my stuff to take home to Minnesota; decide if I'm bringing my car or if I'll leave it and use one of my parents'; if taking my car, find someone to drive from CO to MN with me; look at forums online to find out what the recovery really entails - pain? fatigue?; cancel gym membership and Comcast; pay all the bills sitting on my kitchen table; talk to the billing people at Mayo - what's the insurance process? what will the appointments and surgery cost? what it typically covered? is there any way to cut it down?; talk to Aetna and COBRA to make SURE it's covered and see how much will be covered; think of ways to stay sane in Minnesota - both while waiting for surgery and while held hostage in bed afterward. That's all so far. Hey now, that really isn't so bad, is it? No. It's going to be just fine; I'm going to be just fine. Close your eyes and breathe, Erica. Inhale. Exhale. Inhale. Exhale. You can handle this. It's really not that much. But still I'm scared. I'm happy that I'm closer to my new life, seizure and medication-free, it's just that there's so much to do before I get there. But the second that I drink that in, soak up the possibilities of that new life like soaking up the sun on a perfect summer day, I can't help but smile. Even as I imagine it, I can't believe it. I'll be free. That's really what it feels like. I won't have to take a huge Ziploc bag full of pill bottles on the airplane when I travel. I won't feel dizzy, see double or walk in a zig-zag pattern for an hour after taking a handful of pills. I won't feel stupid when someone asks me a question I can't remember the answer to; I'll remember where someone is on vacation, or what someone's last name is, or which college my friend attended. I won't be so tired. My whole life I've never felt totally awake; some part of me is always tired. I'm always tired. When I was working in sales and had to be bright and cheery all day, I went through phases where I drank six cups of coffee and two Red Bulls in a day. I honestly can't imagine what it will feel like to be awake; to know the absence of the familiar call of sleep. It all makes me smile out loud. I can't help it! I change my worries from a wall to a staircase - a staircase leading to my daydream.

November, 2010

## One of Those Days

Today has been the kind of day that reminds me why I'm doing this. All day I've been having both side effects and seizures. I couldn't tell you how many seizures I've had, cause I couldn't keep track. This morning, I had a 10am coffee meet and greet, and I looked like a well dressed drunkard, stumbling as I followed a zig zag path toward a very welcoming chair.

It's embarrassing when you can't walk straight and have to hold on to every table, railing or wall to stay upright and make it to your destination.

Unfortunately, as soon as the side effects are gone and the world is no longer double, the dirt beneath my feet is no longer tilting and my stomach stops rejecting everything that tries to enter it, it's time to take my next dose. That's what happens on "one of those days". It doesn't end with a cold beer, the way one of those days should, it ends with a 6:30pm bedtime.

I hate beyond hate to complain, but sometimes it's helpful for me to see out loud a reminder - a note of encouragement - of the reason behind my upcoming voyage into my head. Literally.


## Boxes

Boxes. Brown, cardboard boxes, flat and empty and looming in piles around my apartment. Soon enough, they'll be full of all of my personal effects. As soon as I finish my now-soggy Frosted Mini Wheats, that is.

"Packing" sits atop the list I've made of Things I Can Control. In a time when the answer to every question is, "it depends," my spinning head is grasping for any constant it can hang on to. The other day, a friend and I tried comically to readjust the tilting umbrella at a coffee shop nearby to shield us from the Saturday sun. After five minutes of, "okay, you hold down that button and I'll try to move it like this" that led to the woman at the next table snapping a picture on her phone as she laughed, we gave up and slid the wire chairs next to each other in the bit of shade we could find.
We started talking, and soon enough my moving came up. I relayed my now familiar, "it depends." What is the consultation gonna be about? I'm not sure. What kind of tests are they gonna do? It depends. When will the actual surgery be? It depends. What are they going to do in it? It depends.

How long will it be? It depends. Everything depends. I sighed and sipped my medium, iced, skim latte. The chairs were short compared to the table, so I had to reach. "Pilates was good this morning," I offered.

"What are you up to this afternoon?"

"I have zumba class at 4:30."

"No. You are not doing two workouts in one day," she stated. Mandated.

I furrowed my brow and contemplated that. "It's fine," I defended.

"No, Erica, it's not. Listen to yourself. How many calories will you burn between those?"

"Maybe 2,000," I estimated.

"Are you going to eat anything close to that?" her inflection made it unnecessary for me to respond. I had a history with not eating, and she knew it. I knew I couldn't answer, "it depends." I couldn't, because I knew that it only depended on me. When I workout, I can feel my body, and it reminds me that my mind has a tether, it's not just floating in the ether of nothing. It's a great feeling. It pulls me back to the ground. How often I go and how hard I work are things I can control. What I take out of my fridge and put into my body when I get home is something I can control. Finally, things depend on me. Things that I can feel; things that take me back to earth. Things that can pull me back into a place I thought I'd left a long time ago: the sickly familiar gnawing, eroding feeling in my stomach as I put mind over matter and skipped another meal. My reflexes quickly put me on the defense and tried to think of excuses I could give her, but before I could say anything, she added:

"If you're not healthy, they won't operate on you."

Her words hit me in the stomach, knocking the wind and excuses out of me. She instructed me to take out something to write on, because we were going to make a list. I pulled out a receipt and she borrowed a pen from the barista. We were going to make a list of things I can control. Healthy, productive things. At the top of the list was, "Packing," followed by the sub-headings of, speed at which I pack; ship or store; label; organize. I can handle that. I'll start on Monday. Today is Monday, and I'm attacking the first bullet point, starting in my bedroom and moving toward my living room. Now I look at the boxes, the messy pile threatening to fall over, and I smile. This doesn't "depend." It depends on me. Just me.

—

I spent the next week separating clothes, books, canned goods, etc. into three categories: boxes to ship home, boxes for Eve's crawl space and things I attempted to stuff into my overflowing suitcase for Hawaii. My family was going on vacation to Hawaii to spend a week in the sun, getting tan and playing in the ocean. I had largely ignored the preparations as I couldn't take the time off work to join them, but now that I was unemployed, I jumped on the sunshine train.

My parents rented a condo by the ocean with four bedrooms to fit the two of them, my older sister and her husband, my two nieces, and me and my little sister. I so rarely get to see my sisters and their families that I would've gone on vacation to the desert and slept on a couch, but I have to say that I'd rather go to Maui.

## Walgreens on Maui?

Sitting on a bright orange chair, the fragrant purple flowers of a lei spilling down from my neck, I am grateful for one thing: my hair curls perfectly with absolutely no effort in Hawaii!

My flight arrived an hour early yesterday afternoon when the headwinds took a day off, giving me the gift of a walk along the beach just in time to see the sunset. Barefoot in the sand, navigating through fellow onlookers, I fell into step with my mom. Easy enough since I'm an exact copy: same height, same build, same brown eyes and same curly, dark brown hair. The sun ahead of us dipped into the ocean, strong magenta rays shooting heavenward through the clouds that framed it. And the rest of the world melted away.

In the quickly falling darkness, we made our way to the hotel bar, alight with tiki torches. I love tiki torches. A table at the edge of the patio opened up and I took the opportunity to order myself a mai tai. No drinking after the surgery, so I gotta make the most of this! The sun was lighting a tetherball game in Asia, so the waves thirty feet from us emitted only sound. My dad found us through the light cast out from the inside of the restaurant that mingled with the flames, just bright enough to see the waitress approaching, but still dark enough to necessitate a cell phone to read the menu. A smile and a hug greeted him and marked our reunion. Sliding carefully back onto the tall stool, being careful not to bump the wobbly table, we filled each other in on the details that don't translate well over the phone.

A mai tai for me, a longboard lager for mom and something pink, served in a martini glass and tasting like amoxicillin for dad ended our tropical cocktail hour, and we headed back upstairs for a late dinner of Panda Express. Perfection reigned supreme until I reached into my backpack and found: no more pills. Everything was in place, extra quantities for a vacation, except one. There were two nights left of one of the key ingredients of my medicine cocktail. Yikes. Though I mostly have myself to blame, I quickly blamed it on COBRA and their exceedingly slow ability to recognize you as a member. Definitely COBRA's fault. Either way, I needed to find a Walgreens on Maui. My Droid 2, brought to me by the wonders of modern technology, quickly searched "Walgreens Maui Lahaina Locations" and found that the universe does in fact love me. My prescription, $1,200 and ready for pick up in Denver, would last me the vacation, but, sadly, was in Denver. I called the pharmacy on Lahaina, and the pharmacy tech who answered the phone was very likely the most helpful Walgreens employee that I've ever spoken to. He checked to make sure it was in stock, calmly explained COBRA's policies and processes, and informed me that my prescription would be ready in an hour. So today, I would like to formally tell Walgreens that they kinda sorta rock my world.

**Waves**

Lush greenery, the kind we don't get in Colorado, crowds every direction I look, save one. The ocean stretches to infinity, interrupted only by two other islands: misty blue, just darker than the sky they strive towards, rising up from the water.

Sitting on the beach, my legs covered in sand up to the knee, I watch my nieces jump and squeal with every crashing wave. I'm working up my courage to try a longboard. Whether I take the plunge or stay in the shallows with my two nieces, I know I'll soon be covered in salt and sand.

At night we sit on our patio, overlooking the ocean and watching the sun set over Lanai as we sip our mai tai's. Conversation spans everything and lasts well into the night. I struggle to keep my eyes open, not wanting to go to bed for fear of missing something. I so rarely see my family that every minute counts.

We've been here five days, and so far I've only had two seizures. Laughter, sunshine and the loud roar of the waves have proven to be the best medicines yet. Stress is confiscated at customs here, just the same as any foreign plants or foods. Drug trafficking would probably be a lesser offense than the creation or transport of stress.

As it approaches noon, the girls' demands that I join them are too hard to resist.

**Three**

I spoke too soon. I spent four straight days in bliss with no seizures, no side effects, but as soon as I drifted off of Maui to cloud nine, I had three seizures today. The first was around lunchtime and came as quite a surprise. I figured it was just due since I'd gone so long without; like a volcano that erupts every 500 years like clockwork. But a couple hours later, I was bringing dishes into the kitchen and started to have a seizure with a glass of water in my hand. "Mom. Take this. Take this glass, mom. Mom, now!". She knows when she hears that tone, that pitch, the slight edge and strong sense of urgency, that she's dealing with something I can't control, and that I need her help right now. She took the glass of water, and my heart sank. I'd thought this was some magical place where seizures weren't allowed. A place to seek epileptic asylum, the same way asylum is sought here by the newly in love, newly married, and newly heartbroken. No such luck. I racked my brain, trying to think if there was anything I'd done or not done in the past 24 hours to earn me this punishment, but I couldn't come up with anything. Since too often it's hard to see ourselves objectively, I asked my ever-vigilant mother what she thought, and she came up with the most obvious suggestion: pills.

Pharmacies across the country have been implementing a policy of substituting generic pills for brand name when they're available. While this can be cost-effective, the patient is often not notified of this change. That can lead to some serious problems. I can't speak for other disorders/conditions/whatever you'd like to call them, but at least for epileptics, a sudden change in medications can cause seizures. I hadn't realized that my Lamictal XR had been changed to lamotragine (its generic) until I got home. That is my own mistake, but since I have taken lamotragine in the past, I didn't anticipate it being a problem. Again, that's my mistake. When I started to have seizures after a long-by-my-standards hiatus, I didn't know what caused it. Fortunately, my very astute mother had a good idea. Obviously, I can't say for sure, since there are so many factors that influence seizures, but the thing that changed in the past day was the kind of medicine I took.


## Communication Skills

I'm sitting in the Honolulu airport, four hours into a nine hour layover. The Honolulu airport is mostly open-air, filled with concrete hallways with missing walls. The sun is setting, making even the tarmac part of the dramatic scene as it contrasts itself against the blue and pink sky streaked with gray clouds. The noise from an industrial drill outside mingles with flight announcements and a Starbucks compilation. They don't offer their Starbucks sort-of-free wireless here, but my phone tethers and has an unlimited data plan, so I'm not worried. My biggest worry is the battery dying, and my biggest irritant is the way the table wobbles every time I take my hands off it. I'm okay with that.

Yesterday, our last full day in Maui, everyone threw caution to the wind, abandoning the spf 30 for the placebo spf 4. After making pancakes with coconut syrup and crushed macadamia nuts, we spent the morning playing in the waves and soaking up whatever last bit of sunburn we could, determined to make our friends back home jealous of our sun-kissed bodies. Luckily my burn isn't very extensive and is localized mostly on my mid-upper back where, despite my Gumby-esque flexibility, my hands couldn't provide full and even sunscreen coverage. Fortunately we had a big bottle of blue, jello-y aloe, which my littlest niece and I raided that night. Overall the trip was fabulous. My mom and I reflected on our favorite parts: I said that playing on the beach was my favorite activity, but the event that sticks out most in my mind was going with my older sister and trying futilely to hush our laughter as we ran to the ocean to skinny dip at 11pm one night. We were almost caught, too: a dog on a walk with its owner saw us and tried to swim out to us! We swam out farther and it went away, as did its owner. Thank goodness! Life's favorite funny memories are so often made up of close calls.

This morning I finished off half of a pineapple with breakfast just as my phone rang. Picking it up and walking out to the patio to get away from the noises of people packing inside, a woman from the Mayo Clinic introduced herself and sounded thrown off guard when I asked how she was. For those wondering, she was doing very well. She was calling because my MRI needed to be rescheduled. Rescheduled? When was it ever scheduled? She was surprised that I was confused, and it was quickly established that there had been a number of tests scheduled for me and that I was completely unaware of them. Good thing she called!

Miscommunications are seldom the fault of one person. In this case, the moving pieces included me, the back office for the online scheduling assistant, the neurology department, the MRI schedulers, the EEG schedulers and the snail mail appointment confirmation department. Lots of cracks to fall through. Thankfully, the MRI techs take a half-day the Wednesday before Thanksgiving, so my MRI, which was apparently to take place at 4:30, had to be moved up to 2:15. I have no problem with that since I've already blocked off the next three months starting that Wednesday. However, I thought that my appointment with the neurologist was for 7:45am. That is no longer true. As of some point I wasn't aware of, the appointment has been changed to 12:30pm. Good thing to know so I don't have to wake my ass up at 5am and drive the hour and a half to Rochester, MN in the snow. Now I know that I'll be able to get a few more blessed hours of sleep, especially since I don't even get to Minnesota until late the night before.

The woman I spoke to this morning, in conjunction with the woman I spoke to an hour later, gave me a little more color on what my life will entail for the next week. I've already got all the flight information, but as that run out tomorrow night, I'm clueless as to the rest. Shortly after my noonthirty appointment with the Mayo neurologist that my regular neurologist set me up with on Wednesday, I'll have the MRI. Then I get to go home. Unfortunately I have an early morning EEG on Friday, so I'll be spending Thanksgiving night in a hotel with my mom, take out spread across the two queen beds, watching a made for tv movie while she knits. Maybe a hotel room isn't quite our usual dining room table with both leaves in it, a card table and the patio table stuffed into the living room, all surrounded by family and friends, and Panda Express isn't a lovingly-cooked turkey, sugared cranberries, maple sweet potatoes, pumpkin and pecan pies made from scratch and all the other odds and ends brought by smiling faces, but more than ever we have a lot to be thankful for. I have a lot to be thankful for. I have my health. I have a warm place to rest my head. I have so, so many people in my life who care about me. I have a wonderful family composed of both blood relatives and heart relatives. I have prayers for my safe passage coming in from around the world. Beyond that, an upgrade to Papa John's is all anyone could ask for.

Friday morning I'll bring my toothbrush to the hospital and settle in for two or three days of monitoring. They'll then most likely reduce my medication to get me to have seizures while I'm hooked up to the monitoring equipment so they can map what my seizures look like and find out where they originate. Beyond that, I don't know what the plan is, but that's a good start.

The sky here has faded to black, and as the sun went to sleep, so did the sound of the drill, leaving Norah Jones to be heard clearly over the wobbling of my table and the slurp of my straw among melting ice cubes at the bottom of the cup. That's my cue to pack up and head over to my gate, where I'll spend the rest of my stay in Hawaii reading a mystery novel and enjoying some Pinkberry.

### What's the Name Again?

Just checked in and am grabbing some lunch before my appointment! The Mayo campus is HUGE, and I'm in the Gonda building, but my mom and I keep forgetting the name and have resorted to calling it the Gonzo, Gonad, Gorgonzola, Gummy Bear, Gumby and Gumdrop building... More to come later!

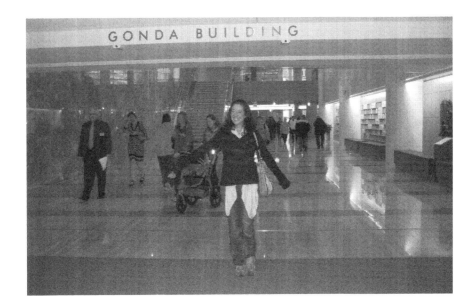

## Zzzzz

I had two firsts in my MRI today: I had a seizure and I fell asleep! I guess we know what happens when I miss my coffee! The gowns they use here are so much easier than the old ones with the ties in the back that keep coming undone and, as everyone who's ever seen one from behind knows, you gots to be sure to wear cute undies cause they're gonna be showcased. The ones they have here have three arm holes, such that you put one arm through each of the first two and the gown wraps around and you put your left arm through the third. That sounds much more confusing than it is... Either way, no ties and your butt stays covered!

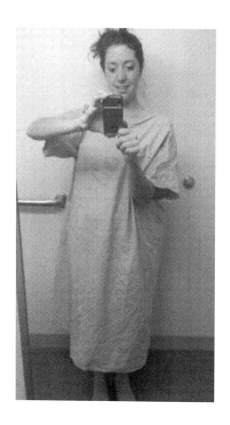

## Plastic Brain Model

I just saw the doctor and was left with a handshake, a "Happy Thanksgiving!" and a pound of butterflies in my stomach. I'm glad they took my blood pressure before. The doctor and his resident were both very nice and very knowledgeable, but not the bearers of good news and assurance that I'd hoped for. He showed me a plastic model of a brain and pointed out where my seizures are. The short circuit occurs right between the motor (blue strip) and sensory (red strip) areas on the left side. The problem is that the brightly painted stripes and chunks are the ones we use most, which is why they are very careful when choosing which between-stripe cracks have extra paint they can chip off. The worry in my case is that they could damage something having to do with my motor and/or sensory functions. The tests that they're going to do on me will determine if they'll be able to pull it off safely. Today is the MRI, and I'll come back Friday for an early morning EEG, followed by one to four days of 24 hr monitoring. God, I really hope I'm a candidate.

## Glue in My Hair

My alarm went off this morning at 5:45, rousing me from my brief sleep at the Comfort Inn on the edge of the Rochester county line. I hit snooze twice while my mom took a shower before tossing off the polyester covers and grabbing my toothbrush and face wash from its Ziploc Freezer Bag. I squeezed out a glob of her toothpaste and looked at myself in the mirror. Today starts step two. My face was still tan from Maui, sprinkled with sun-revealed freckles. My hair was matted from the night's sleep and my loose pajama pants hung from my waist. This is it. It's all becoming real. Months of planning, researching and dreaming are starting to solidify, finding shape from the fog. I took a shower and washed my hair for the last time before it's covered in medical glue. The hotel bathroom's wall mounted hairdryer was surprisingly powerful and made a quick job of transforming my wet hair into a ball of frizz. At 6:30 we grabbed our bags and headed out into the cold Rochester morning.

By 7am I made it to the check-in desk and by 7:10 I had been escorted to one of the EEG testing rooms. I sat in the chair by the lead station and tilted my head back, forth and sideways while the tech measured, glued on electrodes, attached the leads and chatted about Denver. She's thinking of moving there.

The test lasted much longer than the EEGs I've had in the past. It was explained to me that more leads (electrodes) would be needed since I would be going into monitoring. I got to sleep for the first 30 minutes of the test, three blankets shielding me from the cold room. I was then shown a picture to look at, a caption to read aloud, told to hyperventilate for three minutes, and finally shown a strobe light at varying speeds. It starts at 8 flashes per 10 seconds and works its way up, faster and faster until your eyes are watering and screaming for it to stop.

After the test, my mom and I stopped at Starbucks, and I drank my blessed venti nonfat latte and had a breakfast of their Perfect Oatmeal, topped with brown sugar and dried fruit, as we relocated to one of the clinic's satellite hospitals. As the maintenance crew began work erecting the hospital's main Christmas tree and distributed the 92 poinsettias, we were shown to my room. I have a tv with cable, OnDemand and a dvd player, two comfy chairs near my bed, which is surprisingly quite comfort-able, a fridge, a sink, some shelves and hangars and the classic hospital table that rolls to extend over my bed. Quite a swanky room. As I sit and type on my bed, the 32 leads coming from my head wrap together and remind me of Jar Jar Binks from Star Wars. Possibly the most annoying character I've ever witnessed. The nurse came in and explained the general daily schedule to me and gave a rundown of what I should expect and how my room works.

The next one to come was the doctor, who said that we'll be decreasing my medication by half starting tonight to try to induce seizures. That combined with my own plan to over-caffeinate should do the trick. After he left, a technician came in to give me an IV, though not attached to a bag, just there as an access point if needed. I gave her my left arm, since my right will be busy seizing. She unwrapped two overgrown Q-Tips, soaked in dark yellow. She swabbed my arm, tied a blue piece of elastic just above my elbow, and started flicking at my veins, trying to find The One. "Okay, just leettle poke now," she announced in a thick Eastern European accent. The needle inserted into my vein was considerably more painful than I'd expected. I started to recite the Fibonacci numbers in my head like I did as a kid when I got my blood drawn, 1, 1, 2, 3, 5, 8, 13, 21... She pulled the needle out and told me that that one wouldn't work and we'd have to try again. Dammit! She went around the bed to her cart to get two more swabs just as another woman walked into the room and asked if I would like to be part of a study. Sure, what is it? The study is a finer examination of the brain done through more extensive EEG monitoring. I could feel my left arm being iodized again but didn't want to look over. Maybe if I don't look, it won't hurt as much. The test would mean adding 44 more leads to my head for a grand total of 76. 76! I told her to bring it on, but was honestly confused about how they could possibly fit that many on my head! I looked left and saw the needle coming toward my arm like Jaws and could hear the iconic music. I asked the woman from the brain mapping test if I could hold her hand. She laughed as she took my hand and asked me where I'm from, how many siblings I have, etc., and while the needle still hurt, it helped.

The woman from the testing group, Sydney, came back a short while later to cover the remainder of my scalp in electrodes. We chatted as she worked about Black Friday and how she woke up at 2:30 to go to JC Penny, Old Navy and Dick's Sporting Goods. When she left, my mom went through the bag of provisions she brought me from her trip to Target: sugar-free Red Bull, Starbucks frappuccinos, granola bars, Bananagrams, a shirt that zips up the front (since I can't wear anything that goes over my head) and, best of all, a little tinsel Christmas tree that lights up when you plug it into a usb port! The soft white lights dance over the tinsel and bring a silver cheer to my room.

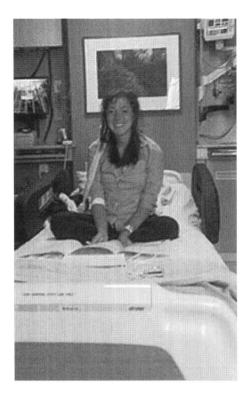

## Combing my Hair and Questioning

The sun splashed against the bricks of the building across the street as I woke up this morning; a reminder to all facing West that it was still there. An EEG tech who looked like Laura Linney came and refilled the electrodes on my head with the special goo that lets the machines read my brain. One by one, I could feel the syringe scrape against my scalp as it wiggled its way through the lead. The whole process took about ten minutes. I think. I can't verify that though, since I've lost all concept of time since being here.

Last night was an eventful one: in twelve hours I had five seizures, more than I normally have in a week. A combination of reduced meds, heavy caffeination and sheer willpower, I suppose. The doctor came in early, shadowed by two residents, and told me that they captured the "events" perfectly and don't think they would gain any more by keeping me longer, so I would get to go home today. He said that the next step will be taking my case to the conference the consultants have every Thursday, which consists of a panel of fifteen specialists, including surgeons and MRI techs, to discuss and see what recommendations they come up with. They're hoping to find some anomaly with the MRI I had done Wednesday. No one has had that kind of luck with my MRI results in the past, but the test I was given is a special epilepsy-finder MRI rather than the standard MRI that's chirped and whirled and clanked above my head in the past. I don't know what it's called or exactly what's different, but I can tell you it was much quieter. The consultants, doctors and techs at the conference will discuss and decide on the best course of action for me. Since my seizures originate from somewhere between the motor and sensory strips, neither of which they like to tamper with, if they don't think that the surgery can be done safely, without compromising any of my motor or sensory functionality, then other options will be explored. Those would include the possibility of an implant - a pacemaker for the brain. If I'm not eligible for that, my regular neurologist will be starting a drug study that I can participate in. If that's the case, I'll likely go see a neuropsychologist as well for the brain equivalent of physical therapy. The butterflies that have fluttered with razor sharp wings through my stomach were appeased at the knowledge that I still have options if I can't have surgery; I won't just be doomed to an eternity of prescription bottles, dizzy spells and fatigue bordering on narcolepsy. The knot in my chest is able to loosen a bit.

In the same vane as there's no such thing as a free lunch, there's no such thing as an easy procedure to extricate myself from the state of epileptic. When the doctor came to see me, he said that the seizures I had while hooked up to the monitoring unit let them confirm that my seizures are originating from the area they had expected. He said that he would bring the case to the conference and discuss surgery as an option, but there he paused. He looked me straight in the eye, an unnerving severity coming through his dark eyes, and told me that this surgery will not be easy. In my case, because of the placement of the origin point, I would have to have two surgeries. The first one would be to open my skull and place electrodes, similar to those I was hooked up to today but much smaller and more sensitive, directly on the surface of my brain. I would then be closed back up for a couple days while more seizures were monitored and recorded so they could see even more exactly where Ground Zero is. The next surgery, a couple days later, would be to remove the electrodes and possibly remove the origin point of my seizures, depending on the results of the "intracranial monitoring." These would be two major surgeries within just a few days. This would not be easy. Afterward I would almost certainly be on medication indefinitely, though much less. I can handle being on medication provided that it's a very small dose that doesn't induce the fog wall in my head and rubbery leg syndrome. But still.

Tonight I sat in a hot bath, combing glue out of my hair for an hour. As I ran the comb through my wet, slippery hair, tugging through tiny globs of dried blue glue, I stared at the shower wall: white and due for a good scrubbing. Two surgeries. I don't yet know if I am, in fact, a surgical candidate, but already I'm conflicted. Am I losing my nerve or am I being realistic? Breaking my skull open twice. Is the prudent thing to run away? Opt for another solution? Would that be smart or cowardly? I really don't know. I want this surgery; I know I do. But I am starting to doubt myself. I've spent the past month and a half romanticizing this amazing new life that will begin after a small blip of a procedure that would really be better described as an inconvenience. Now I hear that twice I'll be wheeled on my back by a team of running bodies in blue scrubs through those iconic double doors that separate the worried people in the waiting room from the unconscious one on the operating table. That'll be me twice. I'm just trying to decide if I'm strong enough for this. Can I do this? Can I really go through with it? How far can I push myself before I break? I don't know. And that's what scares me. I really don't know if I am strong enough. I don't say that from insecurity, I just don't know what my limits are and don't want to do something stupid for the sake of doing it.

When the scalding water became luke warm and the drops on my arms began to give me goosebumps, I rinsed out the remaining conditioner and dried off. Two hours later, I'm still picking at glue, and I'm still questioning myself. Would I really be able to back down after I've come this far? I'd be surprised if I could answer yes.

## False Start

My heart was beating fast as I stood on the starting block, right foot just forward of left. The stands were full of proud parents and reluctant siblings, all stretching their necks to see their contestant. My teammates were right behind me, biting back the cheers that strained to burst out at the sound of the horn. "Take your mark!" I bent forward and grabbed the edge of the block. My meet suit was two sized too small, as was the standard rule for meet suits. I shrugged my shoulders against the black straps that dug into them.

Two blocks down was another girl in a black and purple swimsuit matching mine. Solidarity. "Get set!" I tucked my head toward my body and watched as beads of water rolled down my swim cap to my forehead and fell into the pool. The rubber cap was tight and made my face itch. I exhaled to calm and center myself. The water was like glass, interrupted only by the red and white buoys strung together to separate us from each other. I took another breath and suddenly the world was slow motion. My legs were rubber. I grabbed tighter on the edge of the block to steady myself, panic rising up when I realized that I was about to fall. My body pulled toward the water, knowing it was the easiest way to break my fall, but I pulled back, knowing that nothing was to break the smooth blue surface before the sound of the horn. I wobbled and wished for the horn to blow, but the sound wouldn't come. I glanced longingly at the pool deck, upside down from my perch, and thought of aiming my fall there, despite knowing full well the foolishness of the idea and the high likelihood I would hurt myself when I landed on the wet tile floor. My peripheral vision was cut off by the plastic Tyr goggles covering my eyes. I turned my head back to face the water, knuckles white but futile against my failing legs, and braced myself for an unpleasant speech from my coach as I tipped into the water three feet below me. My heart sank when I heard the false start horn through the water.

When I came up the natatorium was no longer silent. The collectively held breath was expelled into curious and concerned murmurings that ran through the audience. My teammates rushed to the poolside, their faces the picture of worry. Are you okay? What happened? Here, grab my hand, I'll help you out.
One of the judges broke through them and looked at me disapprovingly. I was disqualified. Ashamed and embarrassed, I started to stand up, but kept my head down. Immediately I was covered in hands and surrounded by angry shouts from my team captains. I was a freshman, they were seniors, which made them infinitely cooler than me and I wanted nothing more than their approval. But the shouts weren't at me. I didn't feel hot spit being shot toward me. No, it was aimed directly at the judge. Let. Her. Swim! I can't believe you won't even let her swim exhibition! She wouldn't be getting any points, she'd just be swimming! The rest of my swimming cap and parka clad team stood up in their corner of the stands and started chanting, Let her swim! Let her swim! The rest of the crowd joined in on

the third round, LET HER SWIM! LET HER SWIM! I looked around astonished, I couldn't believe it. All of this, for me? But I got disqualified! I let my team down! Why are they chanting for me?

The judge gave in and the whole natatorium cheered, whooping and clapping their approval. Still a little embarrassed, but growing with confidence and brimming with pride for my team, my team that fights for each other and wins, I climbed the block a second time, took my mark, got set, and swam.

It's been three days since I was released from the hospital and told that if I'm eligible, there will be two major surgeries, not one. I've spent the time nervous and torn. Two? Can I really do two surgeries? Am I strong enough, emotionally, to do that to myself? I've thought about dropping it, dropping the idea of surgery and looking into an implant, instead. The doctor made it sound easier and safer. Maybe I've been too gung ho about this whole brain surgery thing. It's true, I've started down the path, especially in my mind, but I could stop, back up and start again. That's fine. A do-over. I false started. Yeah...

No. I false started when I assumed that I would go home to Minnesota, have one minor surgery, an easy recovery and get back to Colorado completely cured. That was the false start. This, here, now, is my second try. This time I know that it won't be a minor surgery, they'll have to open my skull twice in a manner of days. And that's if I'm a candidate, which I won't know until Thursday. But there's a natatorium's worth of people who have my back. I'm on my second start, though definitely not swimming exhibition, and I'm nervous, I'm scared, I'm not always very sure of myself, but I'm doing my damnedest not to waver. Maybe I'll find that I'm not strong enough to do this, no matter whether it's surgery, a surgical implant or medication adjustments, but I don't have to be. My natatorium, my teammates, are strong. As long as I have them, I can do anything. I've come too far to chicken out and go back. Too far to settle for anything but my best shot.

So I guess that's that. I'm gonna do this.

December, 2010

## Still Waiting

No word today from the doctor. My doctor took my case to Mayo's weekly conference today to discuss my possible surgery with his colleagues and come up with the best course of action for me. He said he'll call me and let me know the verdict, so hopefully I'll hear from him tomorrow.

Last night I couldn't sleep and was having bad side effects; I had to hold on to the hallway wall to walk to the bathroom and steady myself with my hip against the sink to brush my teeth. I felt nauseous, but willed myself not to throw up because I'd just taken my pills. Twice I woke up in a cold sweat. I got up, grabbed a new t-shirt and sweatpants from the drawer, and threw the ones I had on in my laundry pile. I kept waking up, checking the clock, and going back to sleep. Woke up, checked the clock, only fifteen minutes had gone by. I went back to sleep. At 9am I finally got up. But when I stood up, I was still dizzy. Side effects shouldn't last that long. There had to be something else. I took my morning pills and made my way back to my bed. I propped myself up with two pillows, because when my head was horizontal the world would spin. I tried to think what was wrong, what was causing this. Who sneezed on me? They'd better watch their back and get one of those SARS masks before I return the favor, I thought. An eye for an eye - sweaty pajamas for sweaty pajamas. But I wasn't sneezing. I had all the markings of a fever, but my temperature read 97.7 F. And then I figured it out.

The day before yesterday, I ran out of one of my seizure meds. It's one that hasn't been particularly effective, so when I picked up the bottle to add the red and white capsule to the pills in my hand and found that it was empty, I didn't worry too much. It's okay, I'll refill it tomorrow and it'll be fine. But I didn't refill it and apparently it wasn't fine. I missed four doses of that medicine and was paying the price not with seizures, but with withdrawal. That's what it was, withdrawal, not the flu or strep or any other cough-induced ticket to miss school and watch reruns of Matlock. So I stayed in bed all day. I would've done the same thing if I were at my own place in Denver, but being at my family's home made all the difference. My sister went to Walgreens and picked up my pills. She sat with me in bed and showed me pictures of our old high school friends on Facebook. My dad woke me up and made me drink water. I took a sip and handed it back to him, but he said I had to drink to here, pointing to the half way mark on the bottle, and gave it back to me. I'd forgotten what it's like to have a house full of caretakers, working together to make me get better. Twenty hours after it began, I'm not at 100%, but I'm much better. I've had two doses of the medication I'd been missing, which I think has helped a lot. By tomorrow morning it should be building up in my system and hopefully I'll be feeling much better. I've never had withdrawal symptoms like this before, and don't intend to again.

I'd like to say that I've learned my lesson and will never miss another dose of anything, but I know myself and I know that's a lie. But then, what point do I need to reach before I can really say that I'll never miss meds again? I don't know and hope I never will.

There's not really a point to this, an overarching theme with a moral at the end, but I can say that having a caretaker there, in the house, who loves you makes all the difference. Withdrawal is rough, but I'm not alone. Someone is always standing by to hold my hand, make me drink water, and bring me food.

I'm cold now, so I'm going to bed. My phone is fully charged though and the ringer is at the highest volume possible so no matter what, I'll be able to answer in case the doctor calls. I'm about to fall asleep on top of my computer, so I'm signing off.

## Before I Drift To Sleep

The days are blurring together now. Each ends with a paperback falling asleep on my chest and starts again with the snooze button on my cell phone alarm. In between, it's a montage of phone updates from Denver, San Antonio, Seattle, Boston, Minneapolis, everywhere; practicing Pilates on my pink yoga mat on the living room floor, between the glass dinner table and the wall-mounted tv that doesn't work; shoveling away the thick blanket of sparkling snow that covers the driveway; checking my bank account balance; wondering what I'm going to do for a living after this is all finished. I wash dishes with glazed eyes. I sleepwalk toward a foggy horizon, making plans in pencil. I keep a running list of questions to ask my doctor when he calls the purple phone that's glued to my side. Still no word. The Conference, where my case was presented and ruminated upon before my surgical candidacy was determined, was on Thursday. My doctor had told me when I was last in the hospital that he would call me with the results afterward, but as my Black Eyed Peas ringtone hasn't flashed the 507 area code that makes butterflies jump in my stomach, I'm planning to call the neurology department tomorrow morning to ask. Almost harder than not knowing what kind of procedure I'm eligible for is not knowing what to expect from my life over the next couple months. I want to have lunch with this friend or that, but there's a chance I'll be catatonic and regarding light with great sympathy to vampires the world round. My parents want to host a party, but they're not sure if they'll need to keep it down and be available to me at the drop of a hat.

As I sit every day and write this, I want to be clear that this is just a transcription of the thought stream that rambles through my head, not a cry of woe. I am by nature a happy person, which has been and continues every day to be my saving grace. It might just be my own paranoia, but I want to make sure it's understood that these words are not typed with an intention to complain about the lot life has dealt me, but rather are strung together with love and care in a journey of self-exploration as I try to wade through my own mind.

With that, I am put at peace, and will read five more pages of the book on my nightstand before I drift to sleep without marking where I left off.


## Corporate Incentives

I called the doctor Monday, but they said that he was to be out all day, returning Tuesday. I've no longer become surprised.

Waiting for a response is like a corporate incentive: they dangle it in front of you - a shiny new toy or a trip to Hawaii - and you know it's a carrot on a string, because the company doesn't want to give it away. You know full well that you probably won't get it, but a part of you sees it there in your email, in a Monday meeting, on a sign on the wall, and believes that maybe this time you will. So even though the rules change every day to make it more and more unattainable, you keep chasing that carrot.

My carrot is the decision come to at the Mayo doctors' conference. Every day I expect less and less to get the call, but I know my carrot exists, scribbled on a notepad, entered in a computer, floating off tongues to mingle in the air, so I keep chasing it, reaching out to grab it every time I hear the starting horn of my telephone.

## You'll Feel Better In the Morning

My freshman year of college, I took a course called Gender and Communication. My professor said that when they feel frustrated and trapped, men get angry, and women cry. I thought of that tonight as I stood in front of the refrigerator in my parents' empty kitchen. I held open the door, looked down at my feet, dark purple toenail polish showing through the prelude to a hole in my striped sock, and steadied my breath. When I lifted my head, the fridge stared back at me; the sanitary light reflected off the clean, white shelves and frosted drawers. Flavorful food a microwave away from dinner was packed into stackable Ziploc containers. Boxes and boxes of all types of meats, vegetables, fruits and dairies but they somehow held no appeal. Nothing did. I supported myself with one hand on the stainless steel door handle, the other on the counter, and said, out loud, "Erica, you have to eat." The food just sat there, as if waiting for me to pull myself together already and pick something. I repeated it, "Erica, you have to eat." The clear containers dared me. "Erica, you have to eat," again and again, "Erica, you have to eat." "Erica, you have to eat." I warred with myself, one fed up half telling me to grab whatever was closest and stop talking to myself like an idiot, the other screaming back, Stop! Don't rush me! I closed the door, I needed to calm down.

The uncertainty, the way I don't have control of anything in my life, easily welcomed back the anorexia I tried so hard to leave behind in college. The problem is that there's no such thing as a "recovered anorexic," it just goes into remission. It's when you're vulnerable, spinning out of control, that you remember that feeling and you want it back. When you can't control anything else, you can always control what you put into your body. It's mind over matter, and you become so proud of yourself for exercising the discipline not to eat. A sense of euphoria comes over you. It's addictive. It's familiar. It's comforting. I wanted it back, but I knew I couldn't let myself have it, so I repeated the familiar mantra: "Erica, you have to eat."

Sitting now, cross-legged on the floor with my computer in front of me, I'm able to pull back and look at myself. I absently notice the mascara dried on my face; I must look like a mess. My life feels like painting with watercolors when you have too much water on your brush: the red line you drew is muddy; your rainbow is dripping. I painted a whole path for myself: I spent weeks researching procedures, rates of success, risk factors, filling out all the right forms and talking to my insurance company to make sure they'll pay for everything, but now that I've gotten here, my straight lines aren't straight, and there are all of these long washed out lapses of time. Forward is a foggy puddle on sketch paper, back isn't an option, and I suddenly find myself backed into a corner of my own design, asking, what more can I do?, and answering, I don't know. I'm just so tired, all of the time. I don't know these days if it's from the pills or the emotional globe balanced on my shoulders like Atlas.

From the floor, I can see myself and reason with her. Erica, you're tired and you need to go to bed. Go get the turkey chili out of the fridge, put it in the microwave, eat it, then go to bed. You'll feel better in the morning, you always do.


## Unexpected Reactions

Yesterday I found out that if I have a surgery to open my skull and place electrodes on the surface of my brain for a few days, there's only a 60% chance that the doctors would be able to find the origin point of my seizures and be able to take it out safely.

When my phone rang at 9:30 that morning, the white numbers that flashed upon the black display began with those fateful digits, 507. The area code for Rochester, Minnesota. My heart didn't even have time to jump into my throat. A stream of milk was pouring from the carton I held onto the bowl of Smart Start cereal below it when I heard the ringing coming from five feet to my left. I tipped the milk back into it's spout, watching to make sure it didn't spill even as I stretched to reach the tinny sound in the purple case. The number registered immediately as Mayo Clinic, where the fate of my head was being decided.

Hi, how are you?, I asked. Um, very well, thank you. He cleared his throat. My dad thrust a pad of paper and a pen at me while I grabbed hold of the nearest chair. The doctor didn't pirouette or sugar coat, he got straight to why he had called. He said 60%, and I deflated. He rephrased it, saying there's a 40% chance that nothing will happen; that the surgery would have been in vain. How could I have been so naive?, I thought. Of course there was a fair chance that I wouldn't be a candidate. I had known that from the beginning, but didn't actually believe it. He went on to explain my other two options: a Vagus Nerve Stimulator - an implant that runs through your neck to your brain - or medication adjustments. Each had only a 40% chance of drastically reducing the number of seizures I have,

40

and almost no chance of eradicating them. I wrote them down in my hastily scrawled notes, but knew I had no intention of trying either. A fairly common side effect of the VNS is a hoarse voice. Everyone has their thing in life that they're good at; the thing they remember when they come across something they can't do. The thing they remind themselves of, At least I'm really good at ___. For me, that's singing. Not being able to sing would kill something precious inside me; I would rather have seizures all day long. As far as the other option, "medication adjustments," I just can't. I'm too tired. I can't put myself through the headaches, the dizziness, the nausea, the exhaustingly infuriating inability to walk straight or talk straight. I just can't do it.

So that leaves me with surgery. I spent the rest of the day talking to the other ends of my speed dials, and they all said the same thing. With no prompting from me, each one immediately and confidently said surgery. Sixty percent be damned. Notwithstanding the cold I've developed in the last couple days, leaving villages-worth of assaulted tissues in my wake, I'm healthy. I've carved out this chunk of time in my life where I have no job and am living with my parents, each part-time care-giver gifting me with full-time support. There's not going to be any other time to be in this situation; if I'm ever going to do this, it has to be now.

I guess instead of answering my phone, "This is Erica," I'll try, "Sixty percent be damned. This is Erica," and see what happens!


**Restless Peace**

The world around me is coming into focus; the blurry, washed out lines of streets, tables, fireplaces, are drying up to reveal the sharp corners and strong brush strokes underneath. But though I notice everything changing, I don't care. I stare dully at a spot straight in front of me, tired and numb. And I don't know why.

I called the hospital today to set an appointment for my pre-op testing. Someone was supposed to call me, but after a day with no word, I figured I'd make the first move. I traveled to, from and through the switchboard, and found the right person to talk to. She looked at my patient files and commented cheerfully on the large number of things to be scheduled. She analyzed the Venn Diagram of the tests I needed, doctors' schedules, hospital openings and diagnostic machine availabilities and gave me my rough itinerary. January 17th and 18th I'll come in for testing. I'll then see the neurosurgeon on the 19th and have the first operation on January 20th. The timing of the second surgery will depend on how long it takes me to have the requisite number of seizures for measurement. I should plan to spend about a week in the hospital, maybe more. She verified my primary and secondary phone numbers and told me that she will call and let me know the exact times for each event.

When I touched the red End Call button and lowered the phone from my face, I felt a combination of relief, peace and frustration. I had dates; I can make plans in pen now. But it's all in January. I have a month to kill. What am I supposed to do for a month? And then, what about the recovery? I had planned on having all of January and all of February for it, then go back to Colorado. Now I'm thrown off. What if I'm not ready at the end of February? Maybe I should plan to stay here longer. I felt the familiar dull ache in my chest that's become the unwanted companion who comes to me when I don't have the answers. I don't know what to say when I'm asked every version of what my plan is, what I'm going to do before the surgery, what I'm going to do when I get back to Denver, when will the second surgery be, what did the doctor say about it, did you remember to ask this question, that question? I field each one with the reflective expertise of a politician, but inside I just scream, I don't know! I don't know the answers. Hardly any of them. The words "I don't know" consumed me, and as I made peace with them I suddenly couldn't formulate the responses that had come so easily before. The thought of it was a tangible anxiety that nipped at me like an oversized mosquito and pulled my brow in on itself. I was so tired that holding a furrowed expression took too much energy. So with barely the sliver of a conscious thought, I gave in to the peace. The empty peace. I wished the dates were sooner, but at least they existed. The relief and the disappointment that flashed quickly melted away. I want to feel the emotions that I'm supposed to feel, but they're just not coming. It's as if they saw the dullness around me and decided to turn around and go home. And I'm left staring at the wall as the sun sets behind the clouds and the work of shadow casting is taken over by the strands of little white lights that wind up the Christmas tree in the living room.

Tonight I'll spend alone in the dark house, silent with snow, turning my empty confusion into peaceful complacency.

## More To Love

I have a problem. The issue with living alone is not neglecting to take out the recycling, but rather a dangerous and inevitable addiction to tv; particularly sitcoms and crime dramas. In my defense, there is a logic behind it: one turns on the tv for background noise, but the listening understandably turns into watching, and finally to a full dvr. However, as much as I love The Big Bang Theory, I found tonight that I can really only handle one episode at a time versus two simultaneous episodes of the time that Penny is locked out of her apartment and gets hooked on Sheldon's video game. A full disk later, I'm still seeing double, but at least I can walk from the couch to the table by myself. For the worst hour of my side effects, my mom had to hold most of my weight against her for me to even stand without falling over. I cut my dinner short because I knew I couldn't keep it down and didn't want to throw up the pills I just took. Now I sit in front of my computer, hungry despite my churning stomach, but unable to walk to the kitchen and fix myself food, and still having seizures.
My seizures and side effects have been getting worse. I've found myself scheduling my day around them. I know that I'll have side effects in the morning, 20 minutes after taking my pills and lasting 30-45 minutes. I also know that I'll have them again in the evening, starting 30 minutes after taking my pills and lasting anywhere from half an hour to three hours. I don't know when it started or why it is, but my condition and quality of life have been deteriorating quickly in the past few months. It confuses and worries me. Why is this happening? What's changed in my life lately? What am I doing wrong? I don't know. "I don't know" has become the "um" from childhood and "like" from middle school: an ever-present line in my vocabulary.

I know it's been difficult, believe me I do, but I try so hard, and often succeed by virtue of my own stubbornness, to see the silver lining. The only way to get through life is to stay positive; that's the way it's always been and I'm sure always will be. Having debilitating side effects in a house much larger than the shoebox apartment I can navigate with a hand on each wall has forced me to rely on other people. Tonight I had to ask my mom to guide me from the dinner table to the stiff, sage colored couch four feet away. I had to ask my little sister to come hand me my blinking phone because I couldn't sit up, let alone stand or walk. After eighteen years, I'm finally beginning to accept that I can't do this on my own. I need help. I don't have a choice but to rely heavily on other people and be okay with that.

While I would rather not see two tv's mounted on the peach wall in front of me, my double vision gives me more Leonard, Sheldon, Wolowitz, Raj and Penny to love. And who wouldn't want that?


## Dates

No, not with a tall, dark and handsome man who likes long walks on the beach and other stale dating profile clichés. The other kind of date: the test, the conversation, the procedure that fills a white space in my calendar. A scheduling assistant in the Mayo neuro department called me. My phone sang the Black Eyed Peas ringtone that I've been meaning to change, waking me from my sweet slumber. Half asleep, I reached over to my night stand, tugged the charger from the purple device and squinted at its screen. When I saw that infamous 507 area code, my heart began to race under my corporate fundraiser t-shirt, and I answered, "This is Erica."

"Hi, Erica, this is [insert name I promptly forgot]. I'm calling from the Mayo Clinic to schedule your surgery." I forced a deep breath that I hope didn't echo over the line. "On January 17th, you'll have a four hour psych evaluation." Four hours? What are they planning on doing? Is there a movie break in the middle? "On the 18th, you'll have an MRI, which will last at least two hours." I wonder what will be different in this one compared to the one I had the last time I was there. "You'll talk to the neurosurgeon on the 19th, and have your first surgery on the 20th."

Wow. Obviously they'd have to schedule a surgery, but somehow I'd forgotten that it's real. This is actually going to happen. On January 20th, 2011. I heard her say that she would mail me a confirmation of the times, so I didn't feel bad that the questions and realities flash-flooded my brain and made her sound like Charlie Brown's teacher.

I know I already told you these dates, but they crept back into me tonight, as they so often do. I drift to sleep, knowing that I'm covered in a blanket of support, my head resting on thoughts and prayers from amazing, caring, loving people around the world. That is how my eyes can close; that is how I dream in peace. I am so grateful to all of you for giving me that gift.

## Let Me Explain a Little

When asked about the surgeries I'm going to have, I usually explain the first one as opening up my skull and placing leads on the surface of my brain to record some seizures that will help pinpoint more exactly where my seizures originate. Now, however, the surgery is becoming more real by the day, so I think it's high time that we all learn more about what it really is.

The first surgery I'm going to have is to place an Intracranial (inside my head) EEG. eMedicine gives a good summary:
"Intracranial EEG recordings, also known as chronic electrocorticography (ECoG) is an invasive procedure that is performed when noninvasive presurgical evaluation has not led to definitive localization of a seizure syndrome and surgical plan. The presurgical team, which includes a neurosurgeon, neurologist, neuropsychologist, social worker, and neuroradiologist, considers all previous accumulated data to determine an appropriate strategy for placement of intracranial electrodes. Any combination of intracranial strips, grids, and/or depth electrodes may be tailored to answer the specific questions posed by the case history and presentation specific to that particular patient, depending on the needs of the patient, experience of the monitoring team, and resources available for use."

What that means is that the monitoring and testing I've done previously hasn't gotten accurate enough results to perform the surgery to take out the origin point of my seizures. The team, made up of every specialist with the prefix "neuro," will decide the placement of the electrodes that will go on the surface of my brain.

"Invasive intracranial monitoring is a diagnostic procedure, designed to identify the site of ictal onset of seizures. Intracranial electrodes are reserved for the most difficult of cases; therefore, one risk of surgery is that the study will end up with a nondiagnostic result. The onus is on the surgeon to question where electrodes should be placed based on the presurgical information available and to consider what other alternative diagnosis should be included or excluded to obtain the best possible electrode placement. The concept that epilepsy consists of a focus that can be removed has evolved into a more unified theory in which the neural network, environment, genetic predisposition and epileptogenic substrate all must be considered during the evaluation of the patient with epilepsy if surgery is to be effective."

This is the catch: there's a 60% chance that after this surgery they'll be able to identify and safely remove the origin point. There's a 40% chance that they'll open me back up, take the electrodes off and send me home. Hopefully I'll be in the 60%.

The next section is on the technical side, so here's my summary: The electrodes are in a grid, the exact size and shape of which is to be decided by the epilepsy monitoring team. The doctors will perform a craniotomy, where they remove a chunk of my skull to accommodate an approximately 8cm x 8cm grid. The electrodes will be placed on the surface of my brain while I'm under general anesthesia (thank God), and stitched to my brain.

Now the gross part. The electrode wires that are tunneled from my brain, under my scalp and exit several inches away from the craniotomy site to decrease the risk of infection. But not to worry, because they're designed with quick-release connectors that will break apart easily if the wires are tugged. Icky, no? As far as the cut skull chunk, or "bone flap", some people freeze it at the coat check for retrieval when I come back for the next surgery, while other doctors prefer keep it on my head.

Cerebrospinal fluid (brain juice) leakage is normal, but they try to avoid it. So, pretty much, it's an icky, gooey procedure, for which I'm happy to be unconscious.

**Scared**

Last night, for the first time since this whole mess started, I was scared. I've been so cavalier up to this point, so confident that I can handle this easily, and it's worked pretty well. I can discuss it with doctors without clamming up or crying, I can talk about it with friends and neighbors without hyperventilating. Most of the time. Yesterday, I spent the afternoon researching the surgery I'm having done on January 20th. I learned about the factors that determine a patient's qualifications; the basis behind it; strip versus grid electrodes and how they're chosen; the initial incision; what to do with the bone flap that leaves a gaping hole in the side of my head; positioning the electrodes and stitching them to the dura covering my brain; trailing the leads through the skull and skin to hook to the monitoring screen; waiting for me to have enough seizures to procure

46

the information necessary for the second surgery. Deciding if I can have the resection during the second surgery. This is a major surgery, not the easy, open-shut case I'd imagined. I'm about to go through a lot. It's going to be very painful, and I'll have a long stay in the hospital. I'll go under the knife twice. And in the end, I might not even be able to have the surgery I want. I know I've done the research, weighed my options and made my decision, but I can picture myself on the gurney, being rolled into the OR, and feeling terrified. I watch myself, see that fear in my eyes, and the vulnerability there pulls at my own heartstrings. All I want to do is take the daydreamed me and hold her, hold her tightly to me and tell her to give me her burden. Let me take it. I'll take care of her. I keep seeing the lights, the blue masks, through her fearful eyes, trying desperately to will herself calm. I saw her all night. She haunted me all day. I want to help her, but then I look in the mirror and see who she is.

## Mom

Guest writer: my mom

Erica has never let her seizures stand in the way of what she wants to do. This makes me proud, and a little worried. Captain of the swim team. Trekking up Machu Picchu with her Spanish class. Adventures that could spell disaster if she had a seizure or altitude sickness. Her doctor listened and told us it was okay, gave her liquid Valium for Peru if she had trouble. She did it all. No problem.

Erica has been very open about her seizures. Always the first to volunteer for Special Differences day and tell her grade school about epilepsy. This blog for example. When I cautioned that some people might discriminate against her, she confidently replied that she wouldn't want to hang out with or work for someone like that anyway.

Erica has carried her "seizure problem" pretty much by herself. At the age of 7 she gagged easily and couldn't swallow pills, so she had chewable Dilantin, which was awful. She taught herself how to swallow pills, practicing on raspberries and M&Ms. Through middle school, high school, college and work, she does not complain though she takes handfuls of pills every day with pretty severe side effects and poor control of the seizures. She's not angry about her situation.

When Erica told me she was interested in exploring surgery, I knew she had hit a wall. Her neurologist and I had gently pushed her the last couple of years to learn about it. Erica wasn't ready. Now she is.

I love having her back home while we go through the preop evaluations. Initially we were very enthusiastic that she might be seizure free and off medication with a simple nip, snip in her temporal lobe. Now we are more realistic. Erica is very methodical, going through the literature and postings from others who have had similar surgeries, updating friends and teachers, writing the blog.

I feel a little like we are going through a rebirthing process. Tackling this medical problem, learning, hoping, hospital and doctor visits has brought us closer. It has given me more opportunities to mother my independent, creative and productive adult daughter - which I love to do.

## Holiday Parking Lot

Dilemma. I'm at the post office mailing Christmas presents and I just got hit with a wave of side effects. Normally that would just be an annoying inconvenience and I would chill in my car for half an hour or so until I could drive, but today my dad's big, green pick up truck that I borrowed is taking up a primo spot in the USPS parking lot. The usual blacktop is covered in muddy snow and jammed with cars full of anxious people trying to mail off last minute gifts to friends and family around the world. And then there's me, standing by the PO boxes, swaying slightly as I try desperately to stand up straight. I feel just as nervous as they because of the behemoth that is my borrowed truck, stubbornly blocking a much needed slot. I would give anything to be able to move it, to drive to my next shopping destination, but I can't. At least not safely. Behind the wheel, I risk crunching into a woman, a man, a teenager clad in mittens, a fuzzy hat, tall snow boots and an arctic-ready jacket. What can I do? My hands are tied. Or, rather, my eyes are crossed. Agh!! I can't help it, I can't make the parking lot a better place, but how am I supposed to explain that to every Jetta or Prius that honks at me? All I can do is plead to my side effects to please pass, please pass, please pass.

## Sugar Cereal

I don't remember much of those first years; memories come as vignettes, muting to sepia as they float back to me through time. The seizures I remember most are the disorienting, frightening ones before I knew what they were.

I was sitting in the old kitchen on a tall, light-colored wood stool that swiveled slightly as I swung my legs right to left, right to left. My big sister had made me an after school snack of one or another sugar cereal sporting a cartoon character on the cardboard box. I remember her cautioning me when I lifted the bowl near my chin so as to avoid both bending forward to eat horizontally and dripping milk onto my lap. She told me to be careful, don't drop the bowl. I was klutzy as a child, I still am, so the warning was warranted.

I scooped a spoonful of the multi-colored puffs and their pinkish milk, but I couldn't get it to go in my mouth; I lost my aim, my control. I felt that feeling again. Just in my right hand, like always, and though it gripped the silver spoon tight, it veered away, out, and tipped its precarious contents into a rainbow waterfall, green, red, orange, purple, all falling toward Earth and splashing on the hardwood floor below me. I stared, horrified, until there was just a sugary puddle five feet under the offending hand. Horror turned to shame, though I snapped my attention back to my neglected left arm in time to catch it from absently spilling the rest of the bowl onto my navy blue school uniform.

Thinking that I had just spaced out and defied her warning by not paying attention, she scolded me as she grabbed a dish towel and crouched down to clean up my mess. I wanted to cry because I'd let her down and because I had another one of those things I'd been having, but I bit it back until I got up to my bedroom. It was probably ten years before I told her the truth behind the incident. I don't know why I didn't say anything right away, but I guess I was scared and didn't know how to explain it or if it was even real. Maybe it was some weird thing I just made up in my mind.

That was just a couple months before I landed in Boston Children's while on vacation and learned what was going on. The scenes after that are much dimmer. I couldn't say why, though I suppose once I knew what the problem was, it wasn't as scary; it lost some of the mystery that frightened me so. Knowledge is power; knowledge is a flashlight in the dark.

## Winter Wonderland

Sitting by the switch-on fireplace, wearing freshly unwrapped pink, fuzzy slippers and waiting for my coffee to cool enough to drink, I gaze outside. I dare not go out, since my cotton t-shirt is no match for the Minnesota winter, but I'm perfectly content looking through the glass of the French doors, despite the lattice that throws its dark brown stain over the foreground. I can't help but smile out loud at the winter wonderland that greets my eyes. The snow covers the chairs on the deck and the table is topped with a foot and a half of powdery, white frosting. Inside, the smells of bacon and egg strata permeate the air and I'm handed a plate of colorful fruits, cut into bite-size pieces for easy sharing. The Christmas music that streams out of my computer speakers from Pandora is interrupted by a woman reminding us to go to Marshalls for their after-Christmas sale and I can hear my mom shouting up to my little sister to wake up and join us. A conspiratorial look, complete with shifty eyes, briefly crosses my face as I wonder where the leftover Christmas cookies are; my intentions are completely pure though - cookies would really help me avoid the side effects that would make opening presents very difficult; clearly.

Breakfast is ready and served, so I sign off by wishing you all a very merry Christmas.


## Somewhere Between Wake and Sleep

I have questions. Legitimate questions about these surgeries, the recovery, how soon can I know if they can do the procedure or not? I get on and off the phone with the doctors and scheduling assistants so quickly that I forget to ask. Even if I have my Question List in front of me, I feel bad taking up their time with my questions. I forget that I have an obligation to myself to ask and learn about the process of having brain surgery. Someone is going to cut into my brain, so I have every right to ask my questions without feeling guilty for taking up their time. I have to remind myself that. Obligation to myself. Valid concerns. Doctors are there to help answer questions. Those three comprise the new marquee in my head. It builds up my confidence in my own thoughts; my timid insecurities are proven wrong. Will I be awake? I know I'll be put under for the whole first surgery, but if they're able to take the short circuit out of my brain, will I have to be awake during the surgery? Does the decision whether or not to wake me up depend on where in my brain it is? Since mine is between the

50

motor and sensory strips, will they need my services in determining where to poke, pull and prod without leaving me sans-functionality? I really hope not. Also, will they take, or can I get them to take, pictures of my brain while it's exposed? I wanna see it! If they do give me a picture of pink, throbbing brain, I'll post it here for all of you. Especially if they find some kind of anomaly, like they take off my skull and my brain turns out to be turquoise, or it's not a brain at all, but one of those head aliens like in Men In Black. That would be pretty awkward: "Funny story, Erica, we opened you up and it turns out you're not actually human!"... Anyway, my new goal is to be more assertive. Not irritating, but assertive.

## Oops, I Did It Again

There is a word that rhymes with truck. Sadly, there come some occasions where there is really no substitute for it; especially when it had that many cameos in my head. However, for the sake of keeping this PG, I will just say truck.

I have a very bad habit of ordering refills for my pills the day before - or the day that - I run out of them. That has caused me problems in the past, despite the number of times it has been prominently displayed in my New Years resolutions. Before my little snafu in Maui, it had been a long time since I'd had that problem. And then there's today. I swear I did log on to the Walgreens pharmacy site and click the two boxes I needed after searching for them in the long list of prescriptions I've refilled there in the past five years, and I did so a few days before I was going to run out. As I hit Submit, I felt very proud of myself, and when I got the email that my prescriptions were ready for pick-up, I felt even more proud of myself for my responsible ways. And then came today.

Yesterday it rained in Minnesota, Lord knows why since it's December, but overnight it all froze, leaving treacherous streets, to say the least. However, I bravely went forth into the danger (with four-wheel-drive, but still), determined to reach the pharmacy and retrieve my pills. When I got to the front of the line at the pharmacy pick up desk, I stated my name and waited for the scrub-clad woman to hand me the rattling white envelope and send me on my merry way. But instead,

"It looks like we were only able to refill one of these."

What the truck?! "Which one?" I don't know why I bothered to ask, since I'm pretty sure I'll be out of both quite soon. Still, she told me, adding that they're out of it and won't get any more until Monday. Are you trucking kidding me??!! I asked if they had any of the generic, since I used to take that and still have a prescription for it. She replied that that prescription is expired. Awesome. Now I have to wait until Monday to get my pills. I shot up a little prayer that I have enough left to last me until Monday, even though I don't think I do. Maybe it'll be like loaves and fishes, where they magically don't run out - it's still pretty close to Christmas, right?

I paid for the one they did have and walked back to my car, kicking myself despite my best efforts to aim at the store. I climbed in, shut the door, and yelled, "TRUUUUUUUUUUUCK!!!!" Quite loudly, but I don't think anyone heard me. I hope. Driving back toward my house, I continued to yell, "Truuuuck!!! Trucking-a! Truck Walgreens and they're stupid pill ordering!!" but not too deep down, I knew that "Truck Walgreens" really meant "Are you trucking kidding me, Erica? You're a big kid now and should not let this happen." Sigh. I knew that I would have to do what I hate doing more than anything: play pharmacist. I'll ration the pills I have left until Monday and hope that it won't be too bad. I'll only miss one and a half pills, so it's really not that bad, but still, missing medications is not cool. For all of you who take meds, don't make stupid rookie mistakes; order your pills well ahead of time.

2011 New Years resolution: order my trucking pills!!

Happy New Years everyone!!

January, 2011

**No Soup, No Spoon, No Satiation**

That was how we entered the hospital this afternoon after leaving my aunt's New Years Day get together. I started having a bunch of small seizures rapid succession. I told my mom, adding that I think I might be Status. Status Epilepticus is the condition where the seizure activity doesn't stop. Like the Energizer Bunny. So she took me to the hospital for a nice tranq dart. I had to ask the woman admitting me if she could fill out the form for me since I'm right handed and my right hand was seizing. Finally I was rolled back to a room with a decently comfortable bed, despite the pillow. There was only a shower curtain separating my distraction-seeking ears from the nurses' station, which was full of chatter. When I got in, everyone who came in was super nice, but I was still seizing over and over, and it was just a little distracting. I found myself wishing I could just hit zero and magically get some Atavan. I was reaaalllllyy hungry, too, and we had soup in the car, but we left it in the car and we didn't have spoons, so I didn't get any until we got home hours later.

They did finally give me the Ativan and my seizures stopped, but I got really sleepy and looooopyy! I keep falling asleep sitting up as I write this. Writing is good cause I keep forgetting how to structure sentences in real time. My tongue feels big, but the roof of my mouth is so tall; like a cathedral. The sides of my mouth are cavernous. My tongue smmmmmmmmmmmmmmmmmmmmmmmk kkkkkkkkkkkkkkkkkkkkkkk kkkkkkkkkkkkkkkkkkkkkkkkkkkkkkkkkkkkkkkkkkkkkkkkkkkkkkkkkkkkkkkkkk kkkkkkkkkkkkkkkkkkkkkkkkkkkkkkkkkkkkkkkkkkkkkkkkkkkkkkkkkfdf. I just fell asleep on the keyboard. A few times. I really want some pie, but it's the middle of the night, so I don't know. I just had a dream that I was Buffy the Vampire Slayer... I don't know why. I'm gonna sleep now. Goodnight!


**Now That I'm Lucid Again...**

I woke up this morning and looked at last night's post and had to laugh. Yes, the Ativan made me really tired, and a little loopy, but it stopped my seizures.

Everything started at 4:30ish yesterday afternoon. I was at my aunt's house for a small New Years get together for our family when I suddenly started having back-to-back seizures. They were small, one to two seconds each, and happened every couple minutes; by the time they stopped the seizures had lasted almost two hours. I have no idea how many seizures I had during that time.

I had my glass of caffeine-free Diet Coke in my left hand cause I was afraid of dropping anything I held in my right. I'd been having seizures for ten minutes when I finally leaned over to my mom, sitting next to me on the overstuffed couch, and told her that I was nervous. She doesn't hear me say that often, if ever, and her face quickly became the picture of concern. "Should we go to the hospital?", she asked me. That seemed like an overreaction to me, I would just wait it out. But ten minutes later nerves grew as it dawned on me that I might be status - where the seizure activity in the brain doesn't stop, even between seizures. Status Epilepticus can be life-threatening if you have generalized tonic-clonic seizures ("grand mal" seizures), but not simple partial, though it's still scary. My mom asked again about the hospital, citing that we don't want my seizures to generalize - hop across to the other side of my brain and make me have a full-body, or generalized, seizure - cause I would lose my driver's license and could maybe even cause a delay with my surgery. At that point I decided to go. I wished a stream of "Merry Christmas!", "Happy New Year!" and "you too!" as I hugged my aunts and apologized for leaving so early. My aunt ran back to the kitchen as we put on our coats, scarves and boots and brought us a to-go bag with the curry lentil soup and the chicken noodle soup we had drooled over as it cooked but that we would now be missing.

I held my mom by the arm as I navigated down the icy walkway on shaky legs. Not for the last time, I saw that going to the hospital was the right decision. My hand jerked in my lap as we drove to the emergency room entrance, where my mom dropped me off before finding a parking place. I walked up to check in and explained my situation to the woman there, hoping that my inability to fill out the information form with my occupied right hand would help illustrate the time-sensitive nature of my claim. She fastened the hospital bracelet featuring my name and birthday to my wrist and sent me to the waiting room. I tried to be patient as I waited to be called by the triage nurse and finally got in what felt like ages later, though in truth it wasn't even ten minutes. My mom went with me and we sat down facing her desk, our backs shielded by a slightly tinted half wall. When asked why I was there, my mom surprised me by cutting me off and hurriedly explaining my background, impending surgery, problem tonight and what needed to be done. The nurse got me into a wheel chair and told us as we made our way to the doctor that her ten year old son has epilepsy too. I felt bad for her son that he has to have this, but it was comforting that she understood.

She dropped us off at a bed in a room with walls that didn't reach the ceiling and a curtain as a door and gave me a hospital gown shirt to change into before returning to her station. We waited, eavesdropping on the patients to our left, who were in town for the holidays. The nurse eventually came in to assess me and said that she'd never heard of multiple types of epilepsy, let alone simple partial. I was shocked and, honestly, very disappointed in whatever training program had landed her there. But an hour later, as I was still having seizures, the doctor came in and told me that she'd never heard of anything like simple partial epilepsy either, and had to ask me to repeat the name several times. I was then disappointed in the hospital. She was nice though, and ordered that I be given Ativan (lorazepam) to stop the seizures. She also ordered an IV of a gallon of water for me. So I lied in the bed under two heated blankets as my seizures stopped and I drifted in and out of a drug-induced sleep. When the IV bag was empty and they were confident that my seizures had stopped, they gave me a couple prescriptions (including one to bridge the med gap I was about to face) and let me go home.

For some reason, no one gave me a wheelchair, so I shuffled down the hallways in socks, supporting myself on mom's arm. My mom who is three inches shorter than me and whom I could snap in half like a pencil. She set me on a chair in the waiting room by the entrance and ran out to get the car from the parking lot while I stared off into space with my mouth half open and likely drooling. I wouldn't be surprised if people felt a little uncomfortable by the hopped up girl with the stupefied look on her face and tan hospital socks that clashed badly with her black skirt and tights. The boots were much cuter, but I figured heels would be best avoided.

We were finally able to fill our growling stomachs with delicious soup and I forget what else when we got home. I had stopped having seizures but was still out of it and very tired, so soon made my way to bed. Though before going to sleep, blogging somehow seemed like a good idea...

This morning I made it to church, and am glad I did as I was able to run into a lot of people I hadn't seen in a long time, but as soon as we left, it hit me how out of it I still was and the headache was still with me. This time, though, it was definitely not the medication or any kind of New Years hangover, but rather I think it was a status hangover. Status

Epilepticus is not good for your brain. I think how I felt today was my brain recovering from the stress put on it yesterday. Normally, I never have any noticeable after-effects from my seizures, but I'm not surprised that the amount of activity yesterday afternoon took its toll on me. A nap and a cranberry scone helped, and I took the rest of the day easy. All in all, the ordeal was quite the 24 hours for us, but I'm feeling much better now. Thank you all for the support and well-wishing!

## Needles and Rivers and Such

Yesterday I went to my first acupuncture appointment. I had never been to one before, but was convinced into it. My aunt has been seeing her for some time now, and in one of her sessions it was brought up that her niece (me) has epilepsy. Surprisingly to me, as someone not very familiar with acupuncture, this woman works with some epileptics. Curious, I tagged along with my aunt one day last week to talk to this seemingly magical woman. I'd been told already of her stunningly accurate intuitions, and I must say that I was not let down. My aunt and I got up from the waiting area to go to back to the procedure room, and it seemed that everyone there knew the tall, glamorous red-head I walked beside; though after twenty five years, I'm no longer surprised that everyone greets her like a dear friend.

The needle room (as I'll call it, though I realize it betrays my lack of knowledge of the field) has soothing, deep red walls and a stool in the corner for the occasional hitchhiker like me. Two acupuncturists came into the room: one man, tall with a disarming smile, and a short, Vietnamese woman who carried with her a kind and knowing aura. Contrary to my visions of a small room with beads and shrines and an old Asian woman with deep wrinkles and leathery hands, the walls were painted solid colors and adorned with a decorative mirror, such as would be found on the top floor of Crate & Barrel or my living room in Denver. When the acupuncturist, Thuy, greeted me, it was with an impeccable Midwestern non-accent and a clip board. As my aunt laid on the table and the man put the thin, silver needles into her back, legs, arms and head, I asked Thuy about her work with epileptics. She began by explaining to me imbalances. Just as some might say muscle groups or chakras, she told me that the body is made up of twelve rivers. Each river corresponds to different parts and aspects of the body. When a river overflows, the land around it floods; when a river dries up, there is drought; when a river stops flowing and stands stagnant, the water becomes muddy and unclean. All these things cause imbalances in the body; her job is to restore balance. Epilepsy is a symptom of wind in places it shouldn't be. The Vietnamese word for epilepsy, when translated, means "bad upper wind", upper indicating the head. I think that's really interesting and very appropriate: bad upper wind. When one has a seizure, there is a wind inside of them, a force moving the air, causing ripples in the water. The wind invades the head, and as it gusts, beating against waves until drops fly upward from their crests, it disturbs the energy of the river, changing its natural flow and causing imbalance. She works to remove the wind and restore peace.

I was enthralled. I wanted to try. I wanted this woman, this Vietnamese-Minnesotan chiropractic acupuncturist shaman, to balance me.

A week later, I came back. I hung my puffy, down coat on the hook by the front entrance and was handed a pen and five pages of forms to fill out by the curly-haired woman at the desk who somehow remembered me. Ten minutes later, I was shown to my room and given navy blue shorts and a pink shirt that Velcros down the back to change into. Excited and nervously giddy, I obliged, tugging my bracelets over my hand and placing them and my earrings, with the backs re-attached, into the inside pocket of my purse. Removing bobby pins and standing barefoot on a carpet are two of the unsung joys of life.

Thuy came back into the room and sat opposite my chair on the white sheeted bed I would soon lie face-down on. We talked for the next half hour about my health history, my dietary habits, whether I like my liquids hot, cold or room-temperature, and my emotional themes from childhood to 4pm yesterday. By looking at me, seeing me walk, and hearing me talk, she knew things about me that I hadn't even realized until she pointed them out. It was like going to a fortune-telling therapist.

I eventually did get onto the table, my face cradled on a paper-covered headrest that I knew would show make-up-tinted face grease as soon as I moved. She proceeded to adjust my back, my arms, my hip flexors and my neck. She used various torture instruments to suction, scrape, pinch and pull me as I pictured how my aunt had looked as they did the same to her well practiced body the week before.

Finally I moved to the acupuncture bed in The Needle Room. By this point I was relaxed, confident and ready for anything. And then the first needle went in. OW!! Despite the fact that it's needles going into your skin, I hadn't thought it would be painful at all. Yeah, I was incorrect. Granted, some hurt more than others. The first needles went into my face. The one in my forehead wasn't bad, but then she put one on each side of my jaw, into the chewing muscles there, and it hurt like none other! In response to my whimpers, she noted to me that I have a very tight jaw, which was why she put them there. She then said the ones in the face hurt the most, which is why she does them first. That was heartening at least. The next needles went into my wrists. These are my spirit points. She told me that I have a lot of spirit trapped inside of me with no way out. She moved down toward my feet, where she placed one silver torture-toothpick in each, to nurture the energy that vibrates in my skin but that I can't seem to harvest. The rest of the needles she placed in my legs and stomach and chest didn't hurt much, but then, I was still focused on ignoring my throbbing jaw. When Thuy finished, she put a small rectangular bag, filled with beads or sand, over my eyes and turned on soft music, wooden flutes and others I couldn't place, such as one might find in an acupuncture room, and turned off the lights as she left, saying she'd be back in twenty minutes.

I focused on my breath, thinking of the singing I used to do and how much time we spent over the years on breath. I focused on the music, thinking of my long ago trip to Peru. I focused on the pain in my jaw and inner elbows, trying to embrace it and accept it like I'd learned in my three week college yoga class. I slapped my mind on the wrist and told it to be quiet already. Eighteen minutes later, I thought to myself that I could do this forever. I was so relaxed and had no desire to go out and face the world. The almost-zero degree weather, the lights, the noises, the conversation I would have to produce. Who would want to do that when they could be on a bed with heat lamps pointed at them and unplaceable music floating its way to their ears? Only a crazy person. Two minutes after that, the door opened, the lights turned on, and I was cut off. Sigh.

Though the light assaulted my eyes and the loss of the heat lamps threatened goosebumps on my feet, I was addicted. I didn't leave the office until I had another appointment set. Thuy and her magic have found their way into what I've started to think of as my team, just like a race car driver has a service team: amazing people from different therapeutic, stress-relieving, strength-inducing fields, working together to get me ready for surgery and get me recovered. Yeah, I've got people.

# 5 AM

I thought when I left sales that my days of waking up at 5 were done, but I guess not! Today, however, is different, because rather than going to sales meetings, funnel reviews and equally painful early morning phone pitches, I'm going to Denver!!

Surgery is coming up quickly - I have to be back in the hospital for testing in just 11 days. Living at home has been nice, but I'm so happy to get the chance to go back and see my friends before going under the knife.

Denver has been the site of much of my emotional discovery and general centering, so it's only natural that such a place be revisited as I prepare for what will potentially be one of the most transformative journeys of my life.

I've been thinking lately about those "how do you feel today?" magnets that have all the different faces - happy, sad, scared, excited - and a square frame that you place over the one that applies to you as you stand in front of your refrigerator. When people ask me how I feel, I wish I could pick up and stretch that frame to fit over "all of the above". That is the equilibrium I've reached after oscillating between each one, feeling like a silver ball in a pinball machine. Now I just feel a steady state of being filled with a block of indistinguishable emotions, like the brown you get when you mix together every color of finger paint, swirling them from the intended spiral of red, yellow, purple and pink, into an M&M chocolate brown. There are small streaks of each color at the edges, but the vast majority seems impossible to divide again.

My goal for this trip is to sit around a table with french toast casserole and scrambled eggs and talk the colors out.

# Realization

It just hit me that I'm having two major brain surgeries in less than two weeks and I'm scared. I'm really scared.

# Weightless

My head feels light. My shoulders feel light. The headaches that have plagued me prematurely have left. My back is sore, as are my arms, legs, and stomach, but it's a sore that makes me smile. I can breathe. I can sleep. My heart feels light. I am back home.

The Surgeries are coming quickly; I'll be in the hospital a week from tomorrow to start my pre-op testing. But somehow the burden that held me, that pulled my tired head down, my eyes staring numbly at my feet, has dissolved, evaporated. The natural reaction to my Houdini act is to say I don't know how it happened, but that would be a lie. I came to Denver to spend a week with friends, talking and hugging and eating and going to Crate & Barrel, all with the intention to sort out my mind. I've spent the last month so tired, all the time. Part of it was the multicolored handful of pills in my palm, but part of it was the block of mixed up unidentified emotions inside of me. I knew they were there, but I didn't know how to unlock them. Fortunately, a Christmas gift of Delta miles, plus the ten dollars or so I forked over to check a bag, bought me a week of 24/7 therapy.

I helped host a brunch where four girls ate french toast casserole and mushroom quiche and talked about our lives and the feelings they provoke.

I went to Pilates classes at the studio that has become a part of me and magically blocks out the rest of the world as I focus on keeping my hips up, my shoulders wrapped, my ribs in, my feet flexed and my leg lifted as I hold a side plank on the toes of one foot and move the carriage back and forth.

I played Wii Dance, dominating the Ke$ha round but failing spectacularly at Michael Jackson.

I told my sublettor who hasn't paid me rent for two months that I'll change the locks and sell his stuff on eBay if I don't get a check before tomorrow. That last one is actually stressful, not relaxing or rejuvenating, but it's teaching me how to stand my ground, which is a valuable skill. Either way, the cumulative effect of the past four days has been to begin unraveling the knot of neglected emotion inside of me. I can feel it slipping open, exposing to me its colors, light and dark, so that I can begin to understand, accept and deal with each one.

I have two days left in this healing place to build my strength and prepare myself for the challenges moving swiftly toward me and stare them down with the gall I draw from the hands supporting my back.

## Dependent

I grew up fast. I had to, I didn't have a choice. Don't get me wrong, I still went to summer camp, I had snowball fights, I played free the bunch (our version of kick the can) until the street lights came on and I had to go home for dinner. I was a kid, but when I turned seven, part of me wasn't anymore. When I went to camp, I had to be sure I brought enough meds and some emergency options. When I went home for dinner, I had to go upstairs, fill a small, paper Dixie cup with water in the bathroom sink and take my pills. I had epilepsy and I couldn't make other people do everything for me. I didn't grow up fast because of a tragedy or living conditions or narcotics or child labor, but I had a disorder and I had responsibilities to myself.

Independence has always been paramount to me. I was the kid who had to push the elevator button, needed to open my own car door and insisted upon buckling my seat belt by myself. When I got my driver's license, it was important to me to go to my doctor appointments alone. Most of my tests I went to myself. It made me feel independent. If I could do it all without relying on anyone else for help or support, then obviously it wasn't a big deal.

So I went to the doctor, I got an MRI, I got a PET scan, I got my blood drawn, I picked up my pills at the Walgreens drive through. And I knew that if I didn't need help, it wasn't a big deal. But eighteen years after it started, I realized that I do need help. It is a big deal. That doesn't mean that I'm weak or needy, though, and it doesn't mean that my seizures have to dictate my life and my choices. I have a presence in my life that takes a fair amount of my energy and a good portion of my finances, but I'm also a twenty five year old. Just like my peers, I can hold down a cool-sounding job that I know nothing about; I can get dressed up to go out to a bar and spend the whole next day on the couch watching VH1 specials; I can lie in bed looking up at the dark ceiling as I realize I know nothing about life and have no idea what I'm doing. They each have their own problems, just like I do, but that's what makes us unique, that's what makes us who we are.

As the day of my surgery approaches, I realize how much my life is going to change. Whether or not they're able to complete the procedure and remove the origin point, I will never be the same. I look at myself, from the inside to the past, and I wonder how the person I see will look in a month, six months, a year. I wonder which truths I'll realize when I'm forced to let go of that self-imposed solitude. What will happen when, for the first time since I needed a babysitter, I'll have to have someone with me every minute of every day. When I'll have no choice but to loosen my grip on independence and fall, like a team building trust exercise, onto a sea of hands. When I finally, completely do so, I'll find what I've feared for so many years: I don't need to do it by myself.

## Fragile

Yesterday I felt fragile for the first time since I started this whole endeavor. Sure, I've felt scared, but until today, not fragile. I figured I was walking a thin line of sanity, but now I find that I'm standing at the edge, teetering. I tighten my core muscles to reinforce my stability, just like they teach us in Pilates, but standing under the Departures board at DIA this afternoon, any passing fool could've seen that I was barely holding it together.

I had a trying morning in a text volley with my recently evicted sublettor, determining what would be the fate of the possessions he left in my apartment when I changed the locks. I packed my things to go back to Minnesota and I packed his things to put in the hallway. By the time I got in the cab, after leaving the last clothing-filled white trash bag outside my door, I was tired, sweaty, exasperated, and had cussed more in a short time span than I have for a while. "Loser" and "deadbeat" had been thrown in there quite a bit, too. I spent the cab ride to the airport on the phone, consulting my sister on how to proceed, even though her ideas were a little more vicious than mine.

We pulled up to the curb, caked in the dried brown leftover from exhaust fumes stuck to yesterday's fallen snow, and the driver muscled my over-stuffed suitcase out of the trunk. I went on autopilot through check-in and security, pulling my laptop out of my backpack and a one-quart plastic Ziploc containing the coconut lotion I got for Christmas out of my purse. I boarded the tram with the awkward recorded voice toward Terminal C, thankful that it was mostly empty, sat down on the bench and pulled out my phone.

Scrolling through my emails, I found a new one from my dad. I started reading it, and my blood drained and was replaced with boiling lava. He was going out of town from Friday until Sunday. He would leave me in the hospital and miss my second surgery. I was livid, but more than that, I was hurt. A week from today I'll be lying in intensive care, machines beeping and whirring around me, wires coming from the surface of my brain, through my skull, through my skin, to connect to a recording device. I'm going to be drugged, I'm going to be seizing, and I'm going to need my dad with me.

I stood under one of the departure guide signs, writing back and fighting the hot tears that threatened my eyes. I stopped, looking up, trying to keep it together. Don't lose it, Erica. Breathe. I hit send and bee-lined to the bathroom, sliding the lock on the closest stall just in time to lose my resolve. My full eyes broke their seal and tears fell down my face. I wiped them away with the back of one hand as the other reached for a square of toilet paper to catch any wayward mascara. I bit back sobs; I didn't want anyone to knock on the door and ask me if I was okay - the kind of thing I might do. Why would he think it's okay to leave me? I can't do this by myself. I know I'm not really by myself, not by a long shot, but I need someone there to physically hold my hand. I forwarded my mom what I had sent my dad, dried my eyes, and left the stall. The cold water of the bathroom sink felt good as it ran over my wrists. I dried my hands and walked to the gate.

I sat down in an empty row of seats, facing out the window to the tarmac. My phone rang, it was my mom. I almost didn't answer; I had finally gotten it together and didn't want to break again, but I slid the green icon across the small screen. "What? I'm about to get on the plane and I can't talk about this now." But she stopped me. "Honey, your dad is leaving this weekend, not next. He'll be back when we go to the hospital on Monday and will be there through your whole surgery." I guess I misread his email. The oxygen I couldn't find before washed through me, even as my anger was slower to fade. How had I not caught that? "It's okay, you're just a little fragile right now; we all are." Fragile. Breathe in, breathe out. We all are. I'm not the only one here. It felt good, relieving, to know that. It's okay. They'll be there the whole time, four hands holding mine. I can't do this alone, but I won't have to.

## Thoughts From a Friend (Eve)

Hi everyone-I'm Eve, one of Erica's (many!) best friends, and I wanted to write a post about what this whole process of Erica's epilepsy and surgeries has looked like from my point-of-view. I'm neither poet nor linguist, but hope that I can shed some light on what I've observed in the 7+ years I've known this amazing girl. I'm lucky that Erica gave me the go-ahead to write a post on her blog. I'm hoping that as she reads it, she won't regret giving me permission :-).

I met Erica, coincidentally, the same day I met my husband. We sat next to each other in choir. I had transferred to Colorado College as a sophomore, and felt like a nervous kindergartner as I looked around, hoping to find a friendly face in the sea of new people. I'm sure it's not a shock to any of you that Erica was that friendly face - and here we are, over 7 years later, the closest of friends.

I remember Erica telling me about her epilepsy. Like many, I naively thought of epilepsy as portrayed through the grand mal seizures that a classmate of mine had while I was growing up. She quickly explained Simple Partial Epilepsy, and I was amazed at how little I knew about this disorder that effects so many people. In college, I would call Erica from time to time and remind her to take her pills. I would take away her 6th 3rd cup of coffee and remind her that caffeine worsened her seizures. I was always worried about her - but that's my nature, and as she reminded me so stoically, "I don't know life any other way than this. For me, there isn't any other way than this." I was always in awe of how well she handled what seemed like a Sisyphean type of load without thinking twice. She once felt bad for having to miss a final because the side effects of her medication gave her double vision, and she didn't want to make her professor feel bad that she had epilepsy.

I remember the first time she mentioned surgery as an option. I was in my car, driving back from grad school during one of our frequent late-night chat sessions. I bemoaned yet again that the increasingly worse side effects of her medications and its impact on her job and quality of life was not fair. "Well," Erica said, "there is surgery. Brain surgery." I remember feeling a pit in my stomach, and almost feeling relieved when she quickly said, "... but I want for them to make it such a common procedure that doctors are doing it in their sleep before I would consider it. It's not an option right now - and I can just switch medications which should help."

By the biggest stroke of luck, I convinced Erica to move to Denver just under two years ago. A friend like her rarely comes along once in a lifetime, and I was thrilled that she moved from 1200 miles away to 1 mile away. It had been a few years since college at that point, and I hadn't regularly seen Erica during that time. I quickly noticed that her side effects and the number of seizures she was having seemed to have increased dramatically since our college days. Doing what she always did, she switched medications - and the process of incredible fatigue and heavy side effects began. Then one morning last summer, Erica called to tell me she had passed out and hit her head on the counter. "How long were you unconscious?!" I screamed, rapidly calculating how I could get over to her most quickly. "I don't know. I mean, I feel a little woozy but I'm sure I'm fine." Much to her dismay, I dragged her to the E.R. where she got a clean bill of health, but a warning from the doc that she should see her neurologist. The side effects continued to get worse and worse. She would sit on my couch and fall asleep at 7 PM, and I'd have to wake her to tell her to take more of the pills that made her exhausted in the first place.

When Erica told me of her decision to have surgery, I immediately felt relieved. I almost forgot that I had originally felt nervous about the thought of her going under the knife - but now, seeing just how much epilepsy controls her life, I fiercely wanted for my dear friend to get her life back. 15 pills a day, fatigue, double vision, and seizures - that's no life. Am I scared about next Thursday? Incredibly. The date is looming all too quickly on the calendar, and I just want to rush to the recovery part, knowing that it's over, and that she's safe, and her life will be better. But I know Erica is one of the strongest people in the world - and I know this is one of the best decisions she's ever made. Erica, I love you so much-and my thoughts and prayers are with you as you embark upon this massive journey.

**As a side note to all-Erica has graciously allowed for me to post surgery updates here and on Facebook. I will be putting up a "Prayers/Good Wishes for Erica" post the night before surgery. I encourage you to leave a comment for Erica so she is surrounded by our love and wishes as she goes into surgery.**


## Talismans

I've been thinking lately about my hospital room - my hotel room - and how I want to decorate it. I'm not thinking red suede hand chair or trendy printed rug (though CB2 had a really cute one in their last catalog), but the term "hospital white" has a legitimate origin. As I'd rather not spend a week living inside of an anti-septic bottle, I want to find ways to turn the rectangular room featuring a lightly-padded mechanical bed slab flanked by boxes and towers of gleaming stainless steel into a haven for healing energy. The people in my life are the most treasured of my blessings. To honor that, I picked up some cheap plastic frames - the kind with no border, just three open sides into which one jams a picture - at Walgreens for the photos I printed out from their picture uploading website. I'll plant them around the shelves and windowsill, though they'll have to be strategically placed by picture layout, since despite the manufacturer's assertion that the same frame can be used upright for tall-way pictures or sideways for wide-way pictures, trying to balance one on its side is precarious at best and will fall over at the slightest disruption in passing air. So I'll do my best to find the appropriately-shaped pictures for maximum chinsy frame stability.

## Ribbons, Bows and Peace

I think I've reached the point where I'm at peace. I've spent so long thinking, talking and writing that I've covered as much as I can think of and ended up in a calm, comfortable place within myself. I know it's not perfect, and it probably won't be, but what is? My emotions change every day as I come across a new question I hadn't thought of and can't find the answer to; a memory of something amazing I've been able to do, like climb the Inca Trail, eat guinea pig, canoe 180 miles through the Canadian wilderness, despite the epilepsy that seems to consume me now; ideas on how to decorate my hospital room; frantically remembering the restaurants I want to go to, books I need to finish and high heels I need to wear before I'm confined to a bed and my eyes hurt. I am a rollercoaster. I let my head fall to the right and roll its way down, to the left, and back again, dark brown hair falling across my face, trying to wring out my neck. Thuy again put her acupuncture needles in my jaw to release its permanent clench and in my wrists to let out my spirit. Somehow in the dichotomy that surrounds life-altering events, my head feels heavy on its shoulders even while my heart feels hopeful and light. My mind swirls between the two, day by day oscillating from dread to hope and back again, but once I accept it for what it is, revolutions around the axis called calm, I find peace.

I spent a long time unable to distinguish my spaghetti junction of immediate reactionary emotions and mistook them for indifference. Not the genuine indifference of simply not caring, but the empty indifference which comes from the blocking and ignorance of self and that lacks the energy to search. People asked me how I felt about my impending whatever you want to call it - fortune, doom, pain, adventure - and I had no idea of the answer. I would say I was a little nervous but mostly excited, though in truth what I felt was a growing anxiety that I didn't feel anything. But what kind of question is, "how am I supposed to be feeling?" That's a ridiculous thing to wish for a solution to. "It's different for everyone", "Well, what are you feeling?". I just wanted to scream, "Tell me what to feel and I'll figure out how to feel it!!" What was wrong with me? Nothing. There was just too much inside of me, system overload, so I did the only thing I could, which was shut down. And there is nothing wrong with that. I am a rollercoaster, and I needed time and space - mentally and physically - to realize that.

I don't mean to wrap this up with a bow and a clearly stated moral at the end, because there isn't one. I feel a deep, cleansing breath permeating my body, but while peace is the dominating emotion, it's not the only thing in there. Not by a long shot. So instead of the perfectly tied and coiffed ribbons arranged on the top of a gift at Macy's, I'll leave you with color coordinated, scissor-curling-friendly ribbons newly cut but not yet tied.

## Psych Testing of Mexican Tomatoes

*11am*
The water fountain is a ceramic brown that once upon a time was a nice touch to the elegant comfort of the hall outside the psych ward waiting room. Today it acts as a magnet for the grey and white braids that hang from my scarf, pulling them into its miniature tide, taking its revenge against whoever dares disturb its decades old sleep. I stood back up, stacking each vertebra and see the drops of water falling from my scarf onto my black puffy coat. I suppressed an ugh since the drips rolled down the vinyl like little clear balls.

I sat back down in my patterned arm chair and joined my mom in what felt like a staring marathon. The elevator door dinged Up, dinged Down, but the only passengers were young parents with kids and old people pushing wheelchairs of even older people, their deep wrinkles contrasting with the smooth rubber of a baby's cheek and betraying the vast jungle of life that separates the wisdom of one from the new curiosity of the other.

I was transfixed by the scene, wondering at the hidden message it tried to illustrate, but as soon as the elevator dinged again, I barely avoided whiplash as my head swiveled back to anxiously see who was deboarding. The woman I was waiting for had told me that she was wearing a white blouse. Blue jeans and black jackets shuffled on and off, but the research assistant with my forms and itinerary was nowhere in sight.

### *11:45am*
The woman in the white blouse rounded the corner with a clipboard in her hand and an eye contact that was pretty sure but not positive that I was Erica. "Erica?" What's her name? What's her name? "Kari?" Kari shook my hand and squatted down next to my carpet-printed chair, handing me three or four signature lines with a side of pen. She gave me the thirty second canned run down of what each form meant and I blithely signed my name, not bothering to read through the actual type. I may or may not have signed away my firstborn, but I suppose I'll find out another day.

Kari handed me my assigned itinerary and quickly went through it with me. I should be at these places at these times for those things. I was glad to get an official copy of my schedule since I hadn't written any of it down earlier and was guessing at the times.

We very soon realized that Kari was an excellent, somewhat-available asset; a white-bloused answer to "I don't know". Unfortunately, it turned out that "I know" is much more unsettling than I had previously thought. The first surgery will be Thursday, but the second won't be until Monday. What they need is for me to have at least three seizures after the first one before they can do the second; however, my surgeon won't be in again until Monday. I was hoping to spend only a day in ICU limbo with a Saran-wrapped brain and a catheter, but even if I didn't have a four day sentence, it might take as long for me to have the requisite amount of seizure activity. Kari said not to worry if I don't have as many seizures as I expect in a short amount of time, because tampering with the head and brain is a major assault to a disorder that is already touchy enough that the switch from a brand name medicine to its generic can double the number of seizures. Another result of cutting off skull is the Marsha Brady Effect: a good old fashioned black eye. Some people's eyes swell up enough that they can't see. The pain will be bad, even with the drugs. Kari counseled that I take the pain meds every time they're offered me (they'll put me on a schedule), since even if my pain is only a five out of ten, if (when) it does increase, it will be much harder to push the number back downward.

Kari left us with the stack of papers and the new knowledge that I'll be lying with Saran-wrap covering my easy-access brain hole and a comically sized black eye for the better part of a week. The elevator light dinged and we stepped inside.

*12:45pm*
The neuropsych tester wore a pink sweater that reminded me of Dolores Umbridge from Harry Potter. Yellow copy paper was stapled to the tack board wall behind her to create a colorful make-shift backsplash beneath the cabinets that overhung her desk. There was a sign that advertised,

"Five Simple Ways to be Happier:
1. When your heart is open, your light shines through
2. [Something else about light and openness]
3. (I forget)
4. Give more
5. Expect less"

The "heart" from number one was actually a little heart that appeared to be colored in with a Microsoft Office font version of red crayon, and I suddenly thought that pink copy paper would've been more appropriate. Maybe they were out the day she moved in.
The next four hours were comprised of a sequence of tasks that are designed to make you feel progressively worse about your cognitive abilities. The opposite of the Marines: our country's finest are broken down and built back stronger, while each neuropsych test starts out easy and increases in difficulty until you simply cannot answer the question, be it because your time is out or you are just mentally deficient. They said at the outset that no one ever gets every question correct, but that just made me think of the lie we're told as children: there are no small parts, just small actors. That is a blatant fallacy, since at the end of the B- grade play, the audience knows who the main character was, but they couldn't care less about the line-less extra who stood in the back because they mouthed off to the director during rehearsal.

I tended to do well with pattern recognition and reciting back strings of numbers, but had more trouble reconstructing a short story word for word. Some tests turned out to be much more challenging than one would anticipate, such as naming as many kinds of fruit as you can in some amount of time. You read this and think, apple, banana, pear, tomato, orange, what is Erica talking about? But when Dolores asks you to say as many words as you can in one minute that start with the letter F, there's only one that you can think of because it's the only one you can't say.

## 8pm

Four stiff, grainy, light red chunks sat on my plate, staring blankly up at me as we both wondered why they were there. The three-salad medley was brought across the mostly empty hotel restaurant and set on our table by the window half an hour after we'd ordered it. An empty beer bottle loitered on the windowsill as it waited to be taken away with its glass, which was now collecting amber foam in the indent at its bottom. After a day of sitting still, our only movement being the lap we'd made through the local mall as an attempt to get some exercise, in the same vein as those people who walk in sweat suits and ShapeUps through the Mall of America, we were itching for some veggies. I got the chicken pear salad, mom got smoked mushroom salad with ranch, and we split the awkward cashew chicken salad that was marinated in sesame whatnot, covered with wontons and served with French dressing.

No matter how good or bad they were, each dish contained the salad-requisite four tomato slices. I didn't have to even touch them to know how pointless they tasted. "These are not locally-grown," my mom stated to me, "They were grown in Mexico and walked across the border and up to Rochester just to end up on my plate. And now I'm not going to eat them; not because I feel sorry for them, but because I hate them." We both laughed. Neither of us touched the tomatoes for the next hour. [To be clear, this was a commentary on how far away the tomatoes were grown, knowing that Mexico is a common produce producer. We do not hate Mexicans, we hate grainy tomatoes. Just to clarify.]

We joked about life, boys I'd had crushes on, why she decided to go to law school and any other bit of potpourri that was just short of related. Once our exhaustion caught up with us, we gave up and recycled the Mexican Tomato joke until the bill came, went and came back again, and we got to go upstairs and fall into bed.

## Day Two

Pennies. The murse, whom I definitely would have hit on were we under different circumstances, flushed the IV he'd just inserted in the vein in the crook of my elbow. He said the saline might produce a metallic taste in my mouth, like pennies. I've never sucked on pennies before, but I suppose they taste like my mouth.

I much prefer having my blood drawn over having an IV. The attractive murse must've had enough of my drooling over him, because he sent me back to the waiting room. I carefully slid my sweatshirt over the bandaged arm and walked back to the waiting room with my call clip, the kind used at Applebee's that comes to life, beeping and vibrating when your table is ready.

Two minutes later I was again called back and left in a small room that was empty but for three rolling chairs and two computers with paper signs taped to the top of the monitors and hanging their warning in front of the screens that they were for fMRI educational use only. I sat mostly motionless in my chair, wondering what education I needed as I fought the sleepiness that was slowly creeping over me.
A friendly doctor with silver hair cut short and a tongue too big for his mouth that showed itself with every "s" he said sat down in my rolling chair's twin. He flipped the warning sign over the back of the monitor and opened up a PowerPoint presentation. A functional MRI (fMRI to those in the know, or those who have seen the PowerPoint) takes pictures not only of the stagnant brain, but of the brain as it completes certain tasks. The images it creates show colors of varying degrees of intensity that correspond with the activity in the brain when you clench and unclench one hand and then the other, tap your tongue against the roof of your mouth as fast as you can, or hold your breath. They had me do each of those for a couple minutes with small breaks between sets. Despite the many pads and screen monitors inside the MRI that are intended to prevent you from moving your head, I fell asleep. I was roused by the voice of the tech coming through the speakers in my Darth Vader cage-mask and gently admonished for falling asleep and moving my head. Oops.

Plus or minus an hour and a half later, I emerged from the massive magnet, minus one unceremoniously-removed IV as well as two patches of hair that were shaven off to place glow in the dark life savers on my scalp (they were also on my forehead and neck) and the spots were marked with blue permanent marker, which needs to stay on until Thursday. So no more washing my face or hair. For a week or two. Nice and greasy!

Now I've got the rest of the day free, so with a cup of Dunn Bros coffee adding its familiar, comfortable weight to my hand, mom and I are off to explore Rochester!

## Hotel Pull-Out Couch

I woke up at seven with a spring digging into my left shoulder blade. I tapped the touch screen snooze alarm on my phone to at least momentarily stop G. Love from telling me that "it's about time to get out of bed," thinking as I rolled to the sunken middle of the hotel pull-out couch bed that hitting a proper snooze button with your palm is much more satisfying. I'd had one of those rare nights where I'd slept terribly; over my twenty five years, I could probably count the number of those nights on two hands. As I sit in front of my computer I stretch my back, lengthening my spine and roll my head forward, left, right, back again, and try to decide if I'm kidding or not when I say that tonight I should pull what I haven't since I was a kid and try to crawl in bed with my parents. Ah, to sleep in a bed.

When my phone came back to life, lighting and buzzing and singing to wake up, I slid the lock on the screen and turned it off. I struggled to roll myself over the spring that coiled down the left side of the mattress, a barrier to any who tried to exit the bed. Like bumpers in the gutters of a bowling lane - the ball can't get out, it just bounces from one side of the lane to the other, never with enough velocity to spring itself skyward and land in the next lane.

Standing in front of the mirror above the sink, conveniently outside of the bathroom where someone was taking a shower, washing their hair (or what's left...) in the way I can't (not that I'm brooding), I surveyed my greasy face bordered by little blue dots protected by squares of textured clear tape, more cloudy than clear because of their thickness. Knowing it was ridiculous, I carefully applied my makeup around the offending blue pylons; first concealer, then a tinted moisturizer, followed by bronzer, eyeshadow, eyeliner and topped off with mascara, despite the fact that without real soap I couldn't get all of yesterday's mascara off last night, leaving me to wake up with dried black chunks holding clumps of eyelashes together. I know the surgeon and preop team really don't care how I look, but I also know that for the next couple weeks I'm going to feel gross, and though I probably won't care as long as I get my pain meds, for now I'd like to feel like I look presentable. Even adorned with lightly shimmering tan eyeshadow, my eyes were puffy and the whites just short of New Year's Day red.

In ten minutes, we'll leave our haven with its floral patterned chairs and poorly chosen elevator carpet and meet the surgeon who tomorrow will cut me open like Hannibal and put ketchup electrodes on my brain. The rising sun looks welcoming as it paints its inescapable rose colored tint over the bare trees and telephone poles, but I know that just as in Colorado, the view from a Minnesota window can be deceiving, so I grab my black puffy coat as I head out the door.

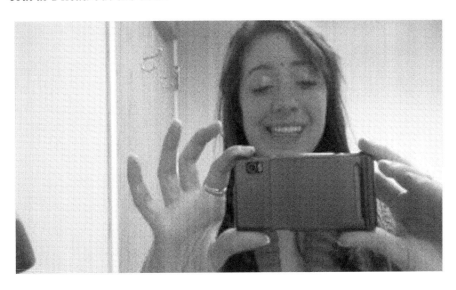

### He's Shaving Half My Head!

We just got out of seeing the neurosurgeon and he said that he'll be shaving half of my head! He has a full head of silver hair, freshly gelled into place. Lucky bastard. The hole they'll be cutting for the craniotomy will be large - a four to five inch diameter. The reason is that they don't know exactly where what they think is a brain birthmark is located. He said what I knew before, that it's right by the motor and sensory strips, so that's what he needs to expose. Whether or not they'll be able to do the resection (take out the seizure origin point) will depend on the location of

74

the birthmark in relation to those strips. The electrodes they'll place on my brain are in a large grid and will be stitched to the dura covering my brain. The scope of these surgeries and the reality of them is slowly coming to me, like an egg was cracked on my head and its insides are creeping slowly down through my hair and over my forehead.

The statistics are much lower than I'd heard before, which was disheartening. The doctor said that sitting in his office today, there's a 25% chance that I'll never have another seizure again. 25%. Maybe 30%, he conceded. I had thought it was closer to 60 or 70%. If they're able to take the birthmark out, then there's a 50-60% chance that I'll never have another seizure. If they can do the resection and I go three months seizure-free and have a normal EEG, that's good. If I go a year seizure free, there's a 10% chance that I'll ever have another seizure, and if I go five years, there's a 1% chance. Pretty amazing. I'll still be on medication for a long time, but hopefully it'll be less. While we're on percentages, here are the risks: there's less than a 5% chance that I'll have infection or a stroke. Both are bad, but it's less than 5%. I'm praying that my fervent praying and that of all the people who are with me can help me avoid that.

The first surgery will be about six hours long and the second one a little less. The average time between surgeries is five to seven days as they wait for me to have enough seizures. They'll likely take my meds down for it, but maybe not. It depends. My favorite two words. After the second surgery, I'll be in the hospital another three or four days. All together, I'll be there ten to fourteen days. Party party!! He said that most of the recovery is done in the first three months, but I won't be totally myself for a year. It does sound like the time between surgeries won't be quite as awful as I've been anticipating, but we'll have to see.

Well, that's about it for now. I'm having a medium skim latte at Dunn Bros as I write, jazz from the overhead speakers, espresso beans grinding and two women planning a wedding at the next table all mixing in the air and making up my background. Next on the schedule is a preop exam, which I understand to be a physical. I've got about twenty hours left with a (mostly) full head of hair to enjoy, so maybe I'll go stand on a street corner and flip it around a little. I'm not allowed to wash it and I didn't bring a flat iron to Rochester, so I'll have to get creative if I decide to try and style it around my blue dots and tape. For now, I'll just deal with the grease and enjoy my coffee.

Until later,
E


**Facebook Status:**
Signed the consent form - we're on! ... eek!
January 19 at 10:33am


Josephine, Stephanie and 2 others like this.
Stephanie Holy cow! I just saw all the posts and read a good chunk of your blog. I'm sending you tons of happy, healthy, seizure ending brain waves, vibes and positive energy! Honestly, and I know I haven't seen you in some time, but I think you could totally rock a complete buzz cut! But what beautiful curls you will be giving up a short while. PS. Your percentages are pretty darn good. Stay strong!
Jillian  See Erica!?!? This is your chance to shave your head, I REALLY want you to do it!!!!
Erica Egge I know you do! No thanks. Greta said her heart is breaking for me, and if they asked her to shave half her head, she wouldn't have the surgery :)
Madeline  Stay strong Erica! I think you'll be hot with a shaved head btw :)
Norma Just remember the old adage, "With a body like this, who needs hair?" Love you!!!
Kate Thinking of you...
Keri We are thinking of you, sweet Erica! You've got the whole OSSC cheering for you!!!! Love you girl.
Margaret  blessing, prayers and love being sent your way!
Jay Best of luck with the recovery, dear. Let us know if you need anything.
Ellen You got this!
Colin As my mom's side of the family would say, God bless you and keep you. And I'm not even religious.


**Too Tired**

I can't. I can't handle this. I'm just so tired. So tired. People keep moving, and talking, and beeping and turning lights on, and I need it to be quiet! I inhale and my lungs pull me back, I exhale and my chest, evacuated of air, falls forward and pulls my shoulders with it. I just can't deal with anything else; I need to focus on me. I'm scared. I'm freaking out. I can't decide whether to repress it or let it out and deal with it. I don't know. But I do know that something inside me, something starting in my low belly and reaching up, wants to scream! I don't know whether its angry, scared or tired; probably all three. I have so many things yet needed of me before I turn off my phone, close my computer, and change into a hospital gown, but I just can't do them. I'm too tired. So tired. I haven't shed a single tear yet. I'm having surgery tomorrow morning and I'm scared and I'm exhausted and a part of me wants it to be quiet and empty so I can break down. Just for a little while. Let me cry, just a little for good measure, and then I'll pull myself together and come back, I promise. Just... just let me collapse. I need to collapse.

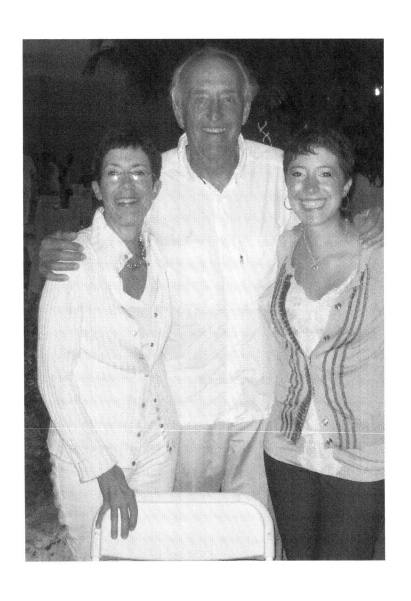

# Part II: Surgery

For my parents for holding my hand, washing my face, feeding me Fruity Pebbles and watching me sleep.

**Leave your prayers and good wishes for Erica HERE**

Tonight, I am asking for your prayers, positive thoughts, and good wishes for Erica. She will be wheeled into the OR at approximately 7 A.M. CST tomorrow morning, January 20th. All day tomorrow we need to be sending her good, healing prayers and vibes. If you are comfortable, please leave a good wish for Erica in the comment section of this post. I know she will feel better just knowing how many of us are wishing her well.

In case you are so inclined-please do not send flowers until next week when Erica is out of the ICU. She can, however, receive non-floral items. Once she is moved into a regular room she will have more flexibility, but the ICU must be free of dust and dander.

I will be in contact with Erica's parents tomorrow, and promise to update this blog as soon as I hear of how things are progressing. We love you Erica-be strong!!!

Comments:
15 comments:

Brendan said...
Good luck tomorrow! It's the year of Brendan, so I'm 100% positive you're going to be fine!
January 19, 2011 7:21 PM

Laura said...
Erica, I love you so much and can't stop thinking about you. I wish I could be there tomorrow morning to give you a swig of m-m-MAGIC m-m-MELLON GATORADE before you start.
January 19, 2011 8:14 PM

Kari said...
Erica--
We are praying for you! Just remember, the waiting is the worst!!
January 19, 2011 9:36 PM

John said...
Dear Epilepsy,

You're going down.... Erica's legit.

Sincerely,

John [Author's note: John and I started dating about three months later and as of the publishing of this book have been together two wonderful years]
January 19, 2011 9:48 PM

Anonymous said...
Erica,

Praying for you tonight and will be at Coco's house in the morning to pray some more! Sending love and good wishes from Redmond, WA for day one of this long awaited journey.

Deb
January 19, 2011 11:55 PM

Gerry said...
Hi Erica, I pray that everything will go great with your surgery, that you will recover quickly, and that the results will show a big improvement in your seizure condition. God bless you!
January 20, 2011 12:49 AM

Sandy said...
GOOD LUCK ERICA! I AM THINKING OF YOU AND YOUR FAMILY TODAY!!

LOVE AND HUGS ALL THE WAY FROM CHICAGO,

Sandy
January 20, 2011 8:39 AM

Anonymous said...
Erica, words cannot express what you mean to me. I know you know that, but sometimes it's nice to be reminded. Being your friend for almost 12 years now (oh my gosh we're getting old) has been one of the greatest blessings of my life.

True courage is something you don't get to see often, but you have shown all of us the beauty of a courageous spirit as you have prepared for today. I wish you the best in all of your endeavors, but especially this one:). I love

you so much!
~Jillian

ps. I'm STILL voting that you should shave your whole head. I've always
wanted to and you actually have a good excuse! Maybe I'll conspire with
your Dad when you're drugged up... kidding... mostly :)
January 20, 2011 9:06 AM

Yumi said...
Ain't no thang but a chicken wang! It was nice knowing you epilepsy, but
you've been voted off!
Love and more love friend!!!!
-Yumi, Adam, & Cali
January 20, 2011 9:56 AM

Susan said...
Is chocolate permitted?
Eve's Mom
January 20, 2011 9:58 AM

Stacy said...
I'm with you in thought and spirit, my beautiful friend. You'll be just fine,
and back in Denver with friends who have missed you sooner than later.
January 20, 2011 2:37 PM

Anonymous said...
Hi Erica! I've been following your journal and thinking of you (especially
today). Sending you the best of healing thoughts from Madison!
-Debbie
January 20, 2011 9:59 PM

Anonymous said...
Dear Erica, I am thinking of you and sending warm wishes, thoughts, and
prayers your way! You are an incredible human being, a strong person, and
a wonderful friend. You have a glowing personality that shines through in
everything you do and it is clearly visible to everyone you encounter. You
are a wonderful presence in this world, and such a kind, caring, genuine
person. I am sending you a big hug and best wishes for recovery!

Much love always,
Natalie

January 20, 2011 11:07 PM

Najada said...
Dear Erica - Karl sent me a link to your journal two months ago. These days I have been checking it daily...I am extremely touched by your strength, positive attitude and braveness! Keep it up! I'm sending you a big big hug and best wishes for tomorrow! I look forward to reading wonderful news.
Najada


## T-1.5hrs!

Well, this is it! I'm sitting on another patterned couch, this one bunches of leaves that, though multi-colored, give an overall impression of mauve. There's a lot of mauve in patterned waiting room couches.

We checked in at the appointed 5:30am and were directed to waiting room two of who knows how many. And me? I'm okay. I really am. Last night I talked to friends: crying with one, praying with another and talking about my new life with a third. I am truly touched by all of the support, prayers, wishes, good luck vibes and healing mojo.

Gotta go get my hair shaved and head cut open, but I love you all and will be back soon.

Erica


## Exam Room

It's getting hard to breathe. My neck feels like a friend who's giving you a neck massage and pulls their thumbs down the sides of your trachea; it kind of hurts, but you don't say anything because they're just trying to help and you don't want to hurt their feelings. My chest is weighted, reminding me of when my hair was three inches longer and fell heavily on it, making each deep breath a push-up for my lungs.

I'm in the exam room, wearing a white gown with little blue circles and dots, two snaps closing it over my bare back. The nurse and tech just came in to ask me every question they could come up with about my medical history, eliciting a rapid fire string of yes, no, no, no, no, yes, from me.

Alone again, I hear the hustle and bustle of voices and carts being wheeled down the hallway marked for employees and escorted patients only. Soon the doctor will come in and listen to my torso move blood and oxygen to its compatriots before clearing me for surgery.

There's a knock at the door. My hands are shaking.

## January 20th, the first surgery

We scurried like mice across the street in the frigid air, hugging the side of the building when we reached it to block out the wind. Refugees under cover of early morning dark, we made our way to the entrance of the hospital. 5:30am. We stomped the snow off our boots and unzipped our jackets to let in the warmth of the heated lobby; my nose was runny. Sitting in his office yesterday after I'd signed the consent form, the surgeon told us to report to the check-in desk at 5:30; my surgery would be at 6am.

The line was fuller than I'd expected, but not particularly long. We had plenty of time. I showed my ID and was directed to the first waiting room. Dad read a forwarded email aloud to us as my mom stared out the window and I blogged on my phone. The jokes weren't funny and we weren't in the mood; mom asked him to read it to himself. It finally hit me that this was real, it was really happening, I'm really getting surgery.

A group of maybe fifteen patients and family members were called from a clipboard to follow a man in blue scrubs into the next level of waiting room. We walked through the hospital halls; the nervous anticipation was palpable and left its scent trailing behind us.

Each patient was shown to their own room and given a gown, a robe, and a plastic bag with a drawstring, labeled, "Patient Belongings", into which my mom placed the folded clothing I'd discarded, my boots and my coat. My dad came back into the room and we sat on pins and needles, trying to make small talk despite our transparency. A nurse came in, a burly but friendly man with a calming demeanor. He inserted my first of many future IVs, smiled at my parents, and began to lead me out of the room. I hugged my mom, I hugged my dad, and told each that I love them. They love me too.

I left the exam room and padded down the hall in my standard-issue rubber-bottomed socks and the breezy blue and white hospital gown, barely tied at the back in neat bows made by my mom's loving hands, and covered with a thin robe. I tugged at the robe as I walked, not sure if I'd put it on right because it seemed to be too loose and threatened to expose parts of me that would be best not seen by the families and friends of other patients who walked past.

The nurse led me into the pre-op/recovery room and onto a bed. A string of doctors came by and introduced themselves to me. They were young, probably residents. The anesthesiologist, a nice man probably in his thirties, joked with me while he explained what was about to happen. He was kind and reassuring. He would be there in the operating room with me. Still, my apprehension was buried in a shallow grave; I'm sure every white coat and blue scrub saw right through my bravery, but they indulged me, pretending not to notice as we chatted.

I was scared. I wanted it to just be over, I wanted my mom, I wanted to be away from here. Why wasn't it time yet? Were they ever going to take me? How much longer did I need to wait? Time lengthened, like taffy or silly putty when you stretch it and it gets thinner and thinner as your arms move farther and farther apart. A few doctors, young, maybe interns, or maybe nurses, I really couldn't tell, stood gossiping around a wall-mounted table surrounded by posters about employee conduct and hand washing. I wanted to listen in, take my mind off the task at hand and find out who'd slept with whom - because obviously it would be the same conversations I watched on Grey's Anatomy - but I couldn't hear.

I was relieved when I saw the EEG tech I'd met back in November when I'd went in for monitoring, Sydney. She was a familiar face, someone I knew, someone who told me she would hold my hand in the operating room as I went under.

Date: Thu, 20 Jan 2011 7:10am
Subject: She's on her way From: Mom

You are such wonderful friends to Erica. She wanted me to be sure to let you know when she was on her way to surgery. I don't think the actual surgery starts for awhile. We were told yesterday 8 or 9am.

Erica engaged the preop nurse in friendly conversation as they went over her preop evaluation from yesterday. The only scowl was when the nurse said she wanted to weigh Erica. I got a photo of her head with hair framing her smiling face which I will send to you. Her blood pressure was something like 105/65. Hardly a sign of anxiety. She said she got her anxiety out of her system last night.

We don't expect to hear any updates for a couple of hours. We will pass on all that we learn. I am so happy you are there.

Becky

Subject: RE: She's on her way From: Jillian

Thank you so much for the update! I am a ball of nerves today and can only imagine how stressful this is for you and Karl. I am so proud of Erica for going for this, not many people would have the courage to do so. Please know that I'm thinking of and praying for Erica today, I've also enlisted the prayers and thoughts of everyone I know. I'll even send a couple your and Karl's way that you can stay relaxed today :).

Thanks again for keeping me in the loop, I don't know what I would do if you didn't!!!

~Jillian

Date: Thu, 20 Jan 2011 7:22am
Subject: She is on her way From: Mom
Erica was her cheery self as we ran across the street from our warm hotel to the hospital at 520 this am. Lots of positive energy. Thanks for your messages and prayers. We won't hear anything for a few hours. But I will keep you updated.

Subject: RE: She is on her way From: Aunt Martha

As I help to wheel our first patient into the room this am, I am constantly thinking of Erica...and all of you. God bless your surgeon and the entire surgical team.

Subject: RE: She is on her way From: Aunt Valerie

Ok. Ok. You were the first topic on our minds/tongues this morning
86

when we rousted ourselves from sleep. Thanks for this note.  Love valerie

## Surgery Update #1

9AM CST 1/20/11

Erica went into Operating Room about 8AM. We are expecting her to be close to out of the recovery room roughly about 3PM today. The surgeon will talk to us then, we understand.

Several things her mom and I would like to share with those who read this blog:

* The number of eyes reading her blog increases daily - to way over 100. This not only happily surprises and pleases her, but she gets a lot of comfort knowing many friends care about and love her.

* Her determination to go through with the surgery is huge - she approached it with unwavering conviction and a smile.

* Last night I (her dad) wanted to chat with her about the 50% (or so) chance that they would not go through with trying to take out the "birth mark", but she cut me off before I barely got started. She only wants to focus on the optimistic.

We so admire our remarkable daughter. Thanks for your love and concern and prayers,

Karl and Becky

On Thu, Jan 20, 2011 at 9:57 AM, Karl Egge wrote:

She went into OR at 7:45, but as of 9:40AM our communicator-nurse said she had not been operated on ... lots of prep work I guess. Understand it will be 4-6 hours of surgery and 1.5 or so hours of recovery before we can see her or talk to the surgeon ... so, 3 to 5PM today.

Erica was so poised, happy, ready, positive about all this. She refuses to talk about the risks, the negatives, the hurts, the implications. Just like a happy soldier.

Becky and I just sitting around in some patient family waiting room trying to find things to do, like poking around on the internet, reading, knitting, responding to emails

Love ya

Karl
From: Paul
Date: 20 January 2011 10:36:00 AM CST
To: Karl Egge
Cc: Peter, Marian, Gladys
Subject: Re: not much to say at 10AM CST

Sitting and waiting with everything beyond your control can't be fun. We are all pulling for all of you guys, especially Erica. Love, Godfather PJ


**Dreaming**

"Mom, it's doing it again," I started crying. What was happening to my arm? Why did it move like this? I didn't like it. I wasn't okay with it. I was scared, really scared. What was wrong with me?

My mom rushed over to me, crossing the carpeted living room of the condo in four strides. "It's okay, honey," she hugged me against her leg, the way only a mother can do. I buried my face in her thigh, my tears seeping through her jeans as she timed it on her watch. Mom was tracking my arm every time it did this. She timed and wrote down each one and how far apart they were.

We had come to Boston for my oldest sister's graduation. It wasn't from college - she'd already done that when I was little - but from some other thing. I think it's called "business school." It was at Harvard, and everyone said that was a really good school. I was really proud of Kendra and told all my friends about her.

The first day we got here, I had five of those things with my arm. The second day, we went to Martha's Vineyard with mom, dad and my other two sisters. Kendra didn't come cause she had to be at school. That day I had ten. The day after that, yesterday, I had fifteen. I was scared. I didn't know what was happening to me. Mom was being really nice, but I could

88

tell she was scared, too.

"Karl, we have to go to the hospital. I'm taking her to the hospital," she told my dad. I was glad when I heard that. I wasn't scared of going to the hospital. Well, at least I was more scared of those things than of going to the hospital. Dad said he'd stay with Coco and Greta - my other sisters. Coco was a teenager and Greta was little, she was just four. I was seven.

I had another one of those things as mom and I stood in line at the desk in the Emergency Room. The lobby at Boston Children's was full of ugly furniture and sick people. There were kids who were coughing, and some kids wearing white hospital gowns with little blue polkadots on them and pulling big, metal stands with wheels on the bottom and a hook at the top with a bag of clear liquid hanging off. The bag had tubes on it that attached to the kids' arms. My brow furrowed. They looked scary. I started to get nervous and edged closer to my mom. I was relieved when the line moved forward so I didn't have to look at the sick kids anymore. Those kids had something else, not what I had. Mine is just in my hand, I'm not sick like them. I'm not gonna have one of those things coming out of my arm, I decided.

The line kept inching forward and finally we reached the desk. Mom told the nurse about the thing that happened with my arm. She told the lady about how she was timing them and I was having more and more and that we'd been to a bunch of hospitals before but no one knew what they were. "Mom," I tugged at her shirt, "Mom," I tugged again until she looked at me, "I'm having another one." I showed her my arm, moving on its own, side to side like a snake. I used my other hand to hold it up to her and the nurse peered over the desk to watch. I could see that she didn't know what it was, either. I deflated as my anxiety and hopelessness overtook the braveness that hinged on the belief that maybe this time they would really tell us what it was and fix it.

The nurse said something to my mom and we went to the waiting room. The chairs were ugly and the couch was too stiff to be comfortable. Mom sat down next to me and I scooted over and nudged her shoulder with my head so she would put her arm around me. The couch was patterned, little square checks in colors that used to be bright but have since faded into neutral purples, blues and greens.

**Surgery Update #2: All going as planned so far**

Hi All-

A quick update as I'm at work. I just heard from Becky that the nurse who is communicating with them said that the electrodes are currently being implanted, and Erica is stable. Just as we had hoped for. Keep those prayers, good vibes, etc. coming! They're working!! I'll update more as I hear.

-Eve


From: Cousin Sarah
Date: 20 January 2011
To: Karl

Hi Unc,

Got an e-mail from my dad that the surgery had not started as of 10 and that you were just reading e-mails...so I thought I'd drop you a note and let you know I was thinking of you and Becky too. You didn't say that you were pacing yet but I'm sure you have/ are analyzing the risks. I have a cutish story for you. Addie and I were talking about Erica (as much as a 3 year old can) and I said that I was thinking of her today and that she had a little germ in her head that the doctor was going to try to fix. I also told her that they were shaving off some of her hair. Addie immediately ran and got some hair accessories (think Cinderella/ Snow White and lots of Pink things) and had the idea that we send them to her so that she has 'pretty hair' and then she got some stickers to put on the other part :). It was pretty sweet.

Again, I'm thinking of you, Becky and especially Erica.

Love you,
Sarah


**Dreaming**

I fidgeted with the white, laminated bracelet with my name on it. It made

90

me feel special cause it meant I was a patient and someone was gonna take care of me.

All the nurses and the other people there were really nice to me. The doctor who saw me earlier was really nice, too. The nurse who we talked to before led mom and me down the hallway. Her name was Erica, too. They told me that I was gonna have some kind of test. I couldn't pronounce the real name, but they said to just call it an EEG. I looked at all the rooms as we passed them, which I knew I probably shouldn't cause it's rude, but I did it anyway. Just before we got to the EEG room I was going to, we stopped as the nurse said hi to a woman who was putting stickers on some man's head. She had a drill that sounded like the one at the dentist's office, but she put it on his head! She was drilling the stickers into his head!! The woman with the thing that sounded like a drill and the man with the stickers on his head must have seen my face, because he quickly assured me that it didn't hurt and no one was drilling into my head, they were just putting on glue.

I sighed, probably out loud, and we kept walking, turning into the room right next door. Erica left us as mom helped me put on a hospital gown and climbed onto the bed table. The gown was white with little blue polkadots and I wondered how different I was from the sick kids in the lobby.

Soon, a short woman who was about the same size vertically and horizontally came in and started talking to us. Mom explained why we came to the hospital and the other tests I've done before, back home in Minnesota. The woman asked me what happened when I had one of those things. I told her about how my hand moves by itself, but I couldn't describe what it felt like, so settled for, "and it has a weird feeling in it." She seemed satisfied.


**Surgery Update #3: Closing her up**

Hi everyone-

I just heard from Becky that they are closing Erica up. They will freeze her large bone flap, and sew her scalp back up. She should be in recovery in about an hour, at which point Karl and Becky will be able to talk to the doctor. They still won't see her for a few hours. Thank you, thank you, thank you for all of your warm thoughts during this scary day.

Date: Thu, 20 Jan 2011 1:07pm
Subject: They are closing Erica up now From: Mom

The nurse just came to tell us that the main part of the surgery is done and they are closing her up. In about an hour they will take us down to the recovery area to talk to the surgeon. A couple of hours after that we can see Erica. Thanks for all your prayers and positive thoughts.

Subject: RE: They are closing Erica up now From: Joe

As a pragmatist, I largely believe in what works. I do believe in prayer and miracles, as God's will has shown me their power in my life.

I am praying to to allow God's healing love to be with Erica and help guide all of us through this passage.
Joe

Subject: RE: They are closing Erica up now From: Eve

Wonderful, wonderful news that she is holding strong and they are finishing up. I'll put this on the blog straight away-I've had people contacting me all day. The whole world is praying for Erica. I sent this to Karl, but I thought you'd like to see it, too (from my mom):

Karl and Becky,

As a parent I can imagine what is running through your minds while Erica is in surgery. So helpless, we often turn to prayer. My prayer is that God gives her surgical team the wisdom and strength to get Erica through this with the best possible results. I don't think that's being too greedy, do you? We're out in CA now and will be offline when Erica comes out of surgery. I've asked Eve to text me with an update.

Erica's friendship has been such a gift for Eve who is a real family person. Away from home, Erica, John and a few other people have become her family away from home. For this Miff and I are so very grateful.
God bless you all,
Susan A.

## Dreaming

The EEG tech told me to breathe in and out really fast. I started, but I didn't like it, it made me feel funny. "Keep going," she ordered. Reluctantly, I pressed on, every once in a while hearing her say, "Keep going, don't slow down." She said the machine was measuring my brainwaves and she wanted to get me to have another one of those things so they could see what happened.

I kept breathing, in out in out, for what felt like forever, even though I felt icky. The lady started to look bored, like she was ready to give up, but my mom kept staring at her watch, flicking her eyes toward the paper that recorded my brain, monitoring the whole process, the whole scene, like a hawk. Suddenly she turned to the tech and said, "You need to put more paper in here, it's almost out. I know these episodes and she's about to have one."

The tech refilled the paper just in time, because exactly like my mom said, I had one. The lady got all excited and leaned out into the hall, calling in a bunch of young looking doctors. I stopped the heavy breathing now that I was having something, but she said sternly, "keep going, keep breathing." Why? I don't wanna, I already got my arm to move and do that thing. I didn't want her to yell at me, though, so I kept going.

People crowded into the room, buzzing excitedly as they watched the needle move on the timely-refilled paper.
Mom looked upset as she watched me and finally told the tech lady that that was enough. I slowed my breath and silently thanked my mom with all the love in my heart as my arm stopped moving and the feeling dissolved into the stale air around me.


Date: Thu, 20 Jan 2011 1:14pm
Subject: She is awake and just fine From: Mom

We don't get to see her for another couple of hours but Erica is awake and moving everything according to Dr M. He said he put about 180 electrodes in her. They are going to do a CT on her way to the ICU to correlate the electrodes with the MRI. When I thanked him for caring for her I told him how committed and optimistic she is about this. He smiled and said he could tell right away yesterday how committed she is. Can't wait to see my baby!

Sent from my iPhone

Subject: RE: She is awake and just fine From: Eve

Wonderful, wonderful news!! I can't wait to hear how she's doing once you've seen her. I have updated the blog to let everyone know she is amazing and out of surgery safely. For once we're praying for her to HAVE seizures-it's so strange! Please send her all of my love. What an incredible woman your daughter is!

Subject: RE: She is awake and just fine From: Jillian

Thank goodness!!! Thank you so much for keeping me posted, I cannot tell you how much I appreciate it. Give Erica a big (but very gentle) hug for me!!!

Subject: RE: She is awake and just fine From: Aunt Valerie

Yippee. This is fantastic news.


**Surgery Update #4: Erica's a rockstar**

Hi All-

Just received word from Becky that Erica is awake and doing well. They still won't see her for a few hours, but the doctor has been in to see Becky and Karl. They placed 180 electrodes(!!) on her brain. We're over this first hurdle of surgery #1 being complete, but the next few days are crucial to figuring out her treatment for the future. For once, we're crossing our fingers that Erica will have seizures. The more quickly she has seizures and the doctors are able to monitor them, the more quickly she will be able to have surgery #2 and be closed up.

# Surgery Update # 5: More news from Erica's parents

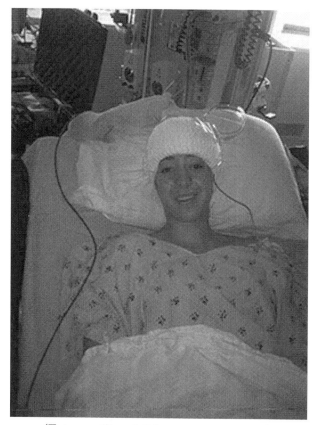

(Erica smiling 2.5 hours post-surgery)

I just got off the phone with Becky, who very sweetly called me to give me more information. She and Karl spent about 90 minutes with Erica, who is still coming out of anesthesia and on a lot of pain medication but her sweet self. She also has a horrible, horrible headache, but that is to be expected. Apparently she was using manners when asking the nurse for things (despite being tired and in a lot of pain).....a girl after this kindergarten teacher's own heart!:-)

As I said before, seizures are the name of the game now. The more quickly she has them, the more quickly her surgeons and neurologists are able to locate the 'birthmark'/seizure origin point and determine whether or not it's safe to operate on it. However, Becky told me that anesthesia is a seizure suppressant, so until the anesthesia is fully out of her system she probably won't have seizures. There is a chance they will decrease the seizure meds she usually takes tomorrow to have more of them occur.

My prayer for her is comfort during this time, for seizures to present themselves to make this between-surgery time short.....and, most of all, for the point of seizure origin to be operable. Erica deserves a new lease on life more than anyone I know-I so hope she gets it. More tomorrow when I have more news to share. Thank you all for your support and love!

6 comments:

Egge Family said...
You're making brain surgery look easy! You look as amazing as you always do. We're cheering you on from Montana. Love, The Junior Egge Family
January 20, 2011 5:59 PM

Kari said...
Great work, Erica!! Hang in there!! You look fantastic!! Thinking of you from Kansas!! --Love, Kari and family
January 20, 2011 7:07 PM

Anonymous said...
That's the beautiful Erica we know. Such a fighter. We send our love!! <3
-Keri and the Route 66 Crew
January 20, 2011 9:24 PM

Susan said...
Thrilled that you have come through this difficult surgery, Erica. Also so very happy the docs are satisfied with the outcome.

So sorry about the headaches. Can they play soothing music for you? Massages? Wishing you comfort soon and good results at the end of this long journey.

Much love,
Susan
January 20, 2011 10:09 PM

Gerry said...
I'm glad she is doing OK.
January 21, 2011 12:36 AM

Anonymous said...
Erica, my thoughts and prayers are with you and I am so glad to hear the

first part of this is over and that you're on your way to healing. Wishing you a very speedy recovery.

Lots of love and good wishes for healing,

Jacci

## Itchy All Over

My groggy eyes fluttered open at the touch of the night nurse's hand on my arm. Sleep's fog still held me as I registered my surroundings: the dark room focused as I adjusted to the the night. A small lamp threw the stainless steel of the bed and machines around me into relief, the white of the walls seeming to glow.

"How are you doing?" she asked. I answered with a half-asleep grunt. The fog around me dissipated into a fine mist and my mind shot open as the sensations of my body hit me full force.

"My head hurts," I offered.

"On a scale of one to ten, what would you rate your pain?"

I don't remember my answer.

"It's time for your pain medication," she assured me, handing over a plastic cup of pills, another of water waiting in her hand.

I swallowed them all easily, a pro in the game no matter the circumstances. I tried feebly to shift my sore body, but I couldn't do it on my own. But the nurse was strong and helped me onto my side, hip and shoulder bearing my weight. "Want me to rub your back?" she asked.

"That would be great, thank you."

"I'm Maria." Her hands moved expertly over my back, soothing the muscles that were stiff from lack of use. Each one sighed gratefully in return, an "mmm" escaping through my lips.

"Could you scratch my back? It really itches."

"It might be from sweat or lotion or something. How about I wash it for you." She moved out of my view into the blind spot that had grown since my head was cut open and wrapped in gauze.

Maria returned with a small, white washcloth that glistened ever so slightly in the cast of the lamp. The cloth felt wonderful on my stale back, caked with poly-cotton residue and dried sweat, wrinkles from my blue and white gown carved into the skin. "Ah, thank you so much. Can you scratch harder?" I asked as I scratched vociferously at my arms and legs. She rubbed the slightly abrasive cloth with more force, but still not enough to satisfy. "Agh, it won't stop. It itches so much!" The uncomfortable tingle covered my body, holding and not letting go, getting stronger by the second.

I pictured a concerned look on Maria's face as she tried to figure out the cause.

There the fog returns.


From: Karl Egge
Date: Fri, Jan 21, 2011 at 9:48 AM
Subject: Erica this morning ... I'd say "fine"
To: Kendra, Coco, Greta

I just stepped out of her room to the family room. She just finished breakfast. Ate agonizingly slow, and Becky helped her. She made it through about 1/2 of raisin bran cereal nicely soggy in milk, about 1/2 way through the 1 or 2 scrambled eggs, 1 bite of 1/2 slice of buttered bread, 2 orange juices and some water (she is thirsty). Electric bed had her sitting close to 90 degrees, but she wanted to get back down. She mentioned she was a bit nauseous and they have a stick w/aroma stuff they wave in front of nose and it sort of denies some of the nausea.

She has a black button/wire pinned to her that she can press to add more pain killer to her IV. So, she is in charge of her pain meds to some degree.

Her right pointer has a gizmo w/light on it that measures through the nail the amount of oxygen in her system, and that goes up on the screen behind her - where also her blood pressure and other vital signs show all the time. Her left hand has the port w/the IV. Her right hand has a port currently

98

tied off. There are 8 or 9 wires coming out of the bonnet heading back to the computers that monitor the 100 electro probes. She has a tube that also comes out and drips bloody fluid slowly into a bag. She has a catheter that empties into a bag in a bucket-like thing under the bed.

Above her bed is a globe that turns out to be a camera trained on her and her vital signs on the screen behind. There are at least 5 if not 8 computer-like screens and key boards throughout the room, as well as oxygen machines, and etc etc. I just marvel at how much money is invested in equipment in that room.

She has a private room. There is a dedicated RN who sits in like a control room at the end of her room and monitors stuff, and comes over and chats or whatever.

Erica tells nurse she has "7" on the 1-10 pain scale. Some of the time Erica's eyes just sort of roll around - like exhausted.

She has not yet had a seizure. That is what we hope she does get in the next couple of days.

Today was -21F in Rochester. I had stopped by Trader Joe's en route down and bought some wine and grabbed a few Summit beers from the basement. Had them in the trunk of my car. Knew yesterday I should have taken out and to the room, but didn't. So, checked this morning and all the things had "popped" and ice-like stuff trying to get out. I put it all by the trash!!!

Love dad

Date: Fri, 21 Jan 2011 11:33am
> Subject: Pretty bad headache From: Mom

Erica ate some breakfast this morning. She is pretty sleepy and doesn't want to talk much because it hurts her head. She is not interested in music or movies so you know she doesn't feel well. The doctors have been in to see her. Probably 4 different groups of them. The nurse thought she may have had a seizure last night so they are going to look at the tracing to see if something shows up. I asked her what I should say if anyone asks why my very pretty, smart, cheerful 25 year old daughter decided to get half of her head shaved and a quarter of her skull taken out.

She said to tell them that it seemed like a good idea at the time. Then she added that it still seems like a good idea. So she is hanging in there. She says to say she loves you and appreciates all your support.

Subject: RE: Pretty bad headache From: Yumi
Hi Becky,
Thank you so much for the emails and phone call. Glad to hear the surgery went smoothly but sad to hear about all the pain. But... I am assuming that is typical? I am looking forward to more updates. Please send her my (and Adam's and Cali's (our dog)) love!

Subject: RE: Pretty bad headache From: Eve

Thank you for sharing Erica's comment of "it seemed like a good idea at the time" - that is SO Erica, and brought a smile to my face :-). You're right, refusing her laptop or Buffy/Bones re-runs means she's definitely not feeling well.

I can't begin to imagine the pain she must be in. It would be great if she's already had a seizure like the nurse said - way to go, Erica!

It must be hard for you and Karl to see her this way - I just know that this is the beginning of her long road to recovery, and hopefully, a better quality of life than she's had. Have they reduced her regular meds yet? Please tell her that the half-shaved head look is "in"-and she has some fabulous hats to wear, too. All my love to you three-what a trooper she is. I'll update the blog in a bit to tell everyone how she's doing on Day 1 post-surgery 1.

## BSU #1
(BSU=Between Surgeries Update)

I heard from both Karl and Becky this morning that Erica remains stable, but has a horrible headache. This is completely understandable given what she's been through. She was able to eat a little breakfast this morning, although it took a long time to eat the little food she did manage to get down. She isn't interested in movies or music-and those who know Erica knows this must mean she's really not feeling well! She says her pain is a "7" out of "10." My favorite part of Becky's update is when she said she asked Erica what she should say if anyone asks why her very pretty, smart, cheerful 25 year old daughter decided to get half of her head shaved and a quarter of her skull taken out. Erica's reply? "It seemed like a good idea at the time" ;-). However, she then mentioned that it still seems like a good idea, so she is in good spirits.

I'll write if I know more, but saw that some were checking the blog today so thought I'd put some info up. Thanks, all, for your love and support!!


From: Karl Egge
To: Kendra, Coco, Greta
Sent: Friday, January 21, 2011 2:40:23 PM
Subject: Update on Erica (just fine)

She is there, then drifts off. Takes lot of pain killers by pushing her button (it has a governor so she can't take more than X in Y period of time), and/ or getting pills. Her spirits are fine.

Becky thinks Erica would enjoy a message from you guys, so feel free to send us an email we can read to her!
So far no seizure.

Not sure I told you she has leg wraps ankle to knee w/hoses connected to air pump - it squeezes in and out periodically. A concern in any operation is a blood clot, and in the calf is major source. E complaining about her right lower leg being numb - the MD says to be expected because some of the electrodes are impinging on the right leg motor signals (or something like that!)

Love dad

On Fri, Jan 21, 2011 at 2:14 PM, Greta wrote:

Kendra and I made a video - let us know if you can get it. I'm gonna try another one!
xo,

G

From: Karl Egge

To: Greta
Sent: Friday, January 21, 2011 4:23:41 PM
Subject: Re: Update on Erica (just fine)
Video works!

On Fri, Jan 21, 2011 at 3:24 PM, Greta wrote:
Can she see/hear my other video? can you?

From: Karl Egge
Date: Fri, Jan 21, 2011 at 3:48 PM
Subject: Re: Update on Erica (just fine)
To: Greta, Kendra

I haven't played either one, because at the moment she is in need of pain med and of nausea med - nicely barks at me if I even talk sort of loud. Knows there are movies of you guys to play - just have to hold off. Her eyes now shut, they just switched nurses so old one introducing E to new one so a lot of yakking and she is just barely hanging on.

Nothing to be alarmed about.

Love dad

On Fri, Jan 21, 2011 at 6:07 PM, Karl Egge wrote:

Read Erica Eve's surgery posts and she was very interested in and liked comments. I wonder if she might try to post tomorrow. She told nurse she was going to do a book about it, and nurse said all of them would buy it!

Below is a photo of Dr. drawing of the "grid" of how her brain is wired with all those probe/monitors.

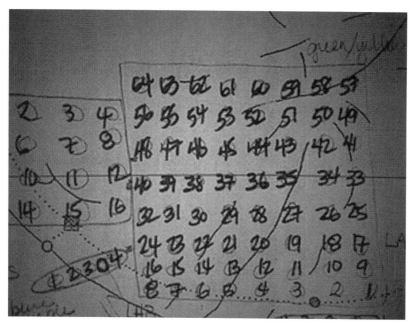

On Fri, Jan 21, 2011 at 4:43 PM, Karl Egge wrote:

Eve,

Erica wanted me to update you.

As for drugs, Becky thinks the fentanyl or dilaudid work better than percocet and oxycodone. There was one spell this afternoon where she was in lot of pain coupled w/nausea. There is a tube (think big lipstick) with some odor that she can sniff and it helps dim the nausea. She has a squirt-like device pinned to her gown that she can push and it gives her more drugs - but it is constrained on how much it can give.

Becky and I are quite awed with how strong and calm she is. She complains of being itchy, which might be due to how cold it is in MN and thus how dry. Becky and nurse rubbed lotion in her, but not quite the thing. At the moment they are rolling her sideways in bed (to her right) so they can put lotion on her back side. Slight chance that the itching is due to the drugs.

Her desired meal for tonight is mac and cheese, oatmeal, and pudding!

She misses you.

Karl

On Fri, Jan 21, 2011 at 8:04 PM, Eve wrote:

Karl-

I cannot thank you and Becky enough for your updates. It sounds like poor Er was in a lot of pain earlier today:-(. I can't imagine how frustrated I'd be if I were itchy all over with the worst headache of my life. I, too, am in awe of her strength through all of this.

I am thrilled to hear that she was peppy over dinner! Did she manage to eat more of dinner than breakfast? I cannot believe the picture of her brain-electrodes diagram. Was it determined that she actually had a seizure last night like the nurse thought?

Send all my love back to her. If she wants to write her book, I'll scribe it for her as she recovers! I'll update the blog again tonight with a picture of the doctor's drawing and the good news that she's feeling more up-beat.

## To the Nines

I think I had just come back from something, but I suppose that doesn't make sense since I never once left my room in the ICU between surgeries. Maybe someone had just come or gone - a family member or the changing of the white-clad guard who watched me carefully from her glass walled-in nurse's observatory box. That's more plausible.

A cleaver had split my head open and lodged itself inside with no plans to leave. Dad sat on the chair at my bedside, his face contorted by worry. Maybe he said something soothing, he probably did, but I couldn't focus, I couldn't think straight; the pain was too much.

"Can't they do anything?" I whimpered, pleading for any kind of relief. Tears sprang to my eyes - no Herculean strength could have held them back. "Dad, help me! It's a nine! It's a nine!" I cried franticly.

Holding my hand, he all but shouted to the nurse behind her partition to do something. Anything.

"I'm sorry, she already took her pain medication. I can't give her any more yet."

My cries verged on sobs. I don't remember if my voice cracked or if I was desperate enough to power through uninhibited when I begged her to help me. "Please." Fat, wet drops slid down my face.

Dad echoed me.

She gave in.


## What Is This Called?

An hour later, though it might have been two hours later, or maybe just twenty minutes, the nurse who'd given me extra painkillers was anxious. I was exhausted, the meds promising the rest my body needed after fighting so much pain. But every time my eyes drooped, the nurse hurried back in to wake me up.

"You can't go to sleep now," she would reprimand, "you have to stay awake." She put on a movie to help - Have You Heard About the Morgans? - but though I tried to watch it, the screen hurt my eyes. I just wanted to sleep. My head was fuzzy, I couldn't think well and I longed for nothing more than to surrender to sweet sleep. But no. The nurse came in in her scrubs and stood in front of the mounted television: "What is this?" she asked, holding up a long, white object with a blue tip.

"A pen," I replied dutifully.

"And what do you do with it?"

I felt silly answering such ridiculous questions, but the words took so long to form out of the ether of my mind. I paused, equal parts annoyed and nervous as I waited. "You write with it," I finally answered.

The nurse looked satisfied for the moment. "Okay. Now don't fall asleep." She turned and walked back to her booth like a sentinel, planning to return in ten more minutes with a stapler or eraser.

## BSU #2: Peppy and Positive

Becky called this evening with a very positive update. It seems that Erica's pain medication has finally started to kick in and tonight she was peppy and happy as she ate dinner. Karl and Becky read Erica the blog posts and comments and she was so thrilled to hear everyone's wishes.

The other good news from Becky is that Erica managed to have some small seizures this afternoon! (I still can't believe I'm excited about Erica's seizures, which until this surgery have made me sad and frustrated on her behalf) The hope is that she'll have more seizures tonight so that her neurologists and surgeons can get the data they need to decide what comes next. This is where things get hazy - my own brain can't really comprehend the specifications that will dictate whether or not the birthmark can be removed... but Dr. M (the surgeon) told Becky he is hopeful that everything will fall into the place that it needs to. If the seizure origin point is closer to sensory than motor in her brain, he will be able to operate. Dr. M says the brain can recover sensory function over time, but cannot recover motor function.* I apologize for my lack of the specifics - when the doctors are able to give Becky and Karl more info I'll try and write it down as I get it to be more concise :-).

I want to take a moment to acknowledge how in awe I am of Erica. I really don't know of anyone else who would be in her position and be as positive, sweet and witty as she is. Her strength provides all of us relief, and that makes this entire scary, un-paved road that much easier to navigate. I am so thankful that she is feeling a bit better, and hope to hear more good news tomorrow.

*I am about the least scientific person in the world, and if I've botched this sensory/motor explanation of the brain I apologize. I was an English major and I teach kindergarten, so I need the equivalent of Brain Surgery for Dummies to help me understand all of this! :-)

## BSU #3: 1 step forward, 2 steps back

It seems like the name of the game when going through/recovering from any medical procedure is accepting the good news with the bad.

1 step forward: Erica had two mini seizures this morning. I'm glad she's

having them! More data=more information for her docs.

2 steps back: Erica is in a lot of pain so far today, and is very nauseous :-(. Some of her aunts were down to visit her today, and said that she was able to chat with them despite being incredibly uncomfortable. Her Aunt Kate reported that Erica will likely see the doctor today and maybe even hear about the next surgery.

I hope to update later today with more steps forward, and fewer steps backwards. Hang in there, sweet Er.

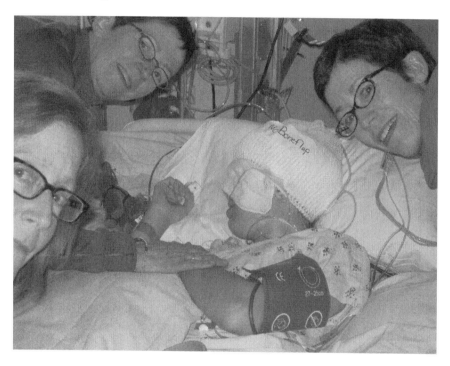

## BSU #4: Surgery Likely on Monday

Erica had a really hard day today. She was in an incredible amount of pain, and not much could be done to help her. She ate very little at breakfast and lunch and was listless most of the day. However, just like last night, Erica pepped up at dinner time. She was able to eat a little and had a good time Skyping with her sister Kendra.

One of the most important updates I can give you right now is that surgery #2 will most likely be on Monday. As long as there are no

107

emergency brain surgeries that come in on Monday morning, the OR is reserved for Erica. At this point, they are still unsure as to whether or not they will be able to excise the birthmark. Of the over 100 electrodes on her brain, they've been able to ascertain which 5 or 6 are located right over the birthmark. Karl explained that on Monday morning they will send voltage to these 5 or 6 electrodes. If the voltage causes her to sense a seizure, good - this will mean they can remove the birthmark before putting on the skull cap again. However, if the voltage causes her arm to move first they will just put the skull cap back on without cutting out the birthmark.

There is a chance I'll get to talk to Erica on the phone tomorrow if she's feeling up to it. I am really looking forward to hearing her voice and telling her how many people are thinking about her and praying for her. Good night for now.

3 comments:

Susan said...
Sending our love and encouragement from CA to our brave Erica. We'll have her in our minds and hearts on Monday and eagerly await Eve's updates.

All our love, Miff and Susan
January 22, 2011 10:44 PM

Anonymous said...
Thinking of you Erica!! Just read your blog - you are an amazing writer!! And what a sweet friend you have in Eve!!! You are in my thoughts and prayers every moment!! My love to you and your Mom and Dad!! Scott sends his good wishes, too!! Mickey

P.S. Can't figure out the "comment as" thing! Forgive the "anonymous" designation!!!
January 23, 2011 12:39 PM

Anonymous said...
I'm sending so many positive thoughts and prayers to you and your family this morning, erica!

I've just met you (through your amazing blog) and you're one of the most inspiring and courageous women i've ever known.

Thank you for sharing your journey, and reminding me of what's important in life.

with lots of love, caroline (kendra's friend)
January 24, 2011 8:01 AM


## BSU # 5: Chatting about tomorrow

I was able to chat with Erica on Skype today! It was great to 'see' her - I've said before and I'll say it again (and again, and again!) how amazed I am at Erica's cheerfulness and up-beat attitude during a really hard time. We talked about everything from the details of what's been happening with her care to the weather, and it made me so happy just to know my sweet friend was doing okay. Her pain was far less this morning than it's been which is wonderful, wonderful news!

What's next? Tomorrow is THE big day. D-day. At approximately 8 AM CST, Erica will begin her "brain-mapping" test. This is what I talked about last night where Dr. W will send voltage to the 5 or 6 electrodes right over the birthmark. Based on this test (which should take a few hours), the decision will be either resecting or just putting the skull cap back on. As I understand it, Erica's doctors feel that if they are able to do the resection, there is a 70% chance that she'll not have any more seizures! She will have to remain on medication indefinitely, but will hopefully be without seizures.

In the chance that they are unable to resect and they just put the skull cap back on, they've already told Erica they have some other ideas that will hopefully help her not have the medication problems and constant seizures she's had up to now. Of course the hope is that resection will work, but the Egges are optimistic that no matter what happens, Erica has options. Despite being in pain and going through an incredible ordeal, Erica knows this was the right decision. What a trooper!

Like I did on Thursday, I'll post updates tomorrow throughout Erica's two procedures (the mapping first, the surgery second) as I receive them from Becky and Karl. Fingers crossed for great news tomorrow!

10 comments:

Gladys said...
Eve, Thank you for updating this blog. Erica is on our minds most of each day. The blog is so helpful. Erica's comfort sounds fine; of course, we're all hoping that the doctors will be able to alleviate her problem significantly.

Aunt Gladys
January 23, 2011 5:57 PM

Anonymous said...
Thank you so much Eve, for keeping us updated. All our love to you, Miss Erica, as we are all thinking about you constantly. You are one of the most brave people I know and I fully trust that all will be well! Sending love your way!!!
<3<3<3 Keri, Justin and the Crew
January 23, 2011 6:34 PM

Susan said...
Dear, Dear Erica,

We'll be checking the blog often on Monday and hoping and praying that your efforts (and the doctors') will pay off as we've all hoped.

Be strong, know that you are loved and cherished by so many who know you; and start preparing for a bright and healthy rest of your life.

Always,
Susan and Miff
January 23, 2011 6:58 PM

Mindy and Jeff said...
We are thinking of you, Erica!! We hope tomorrow goes really well for you. Stay strong & upbeat. :)

Hugs!
January 23, 2011 7:16 PM

Gerry said...
I've been reading this blog everyday, and am hoping that Erica gets good news :)

January 23, 2011 8:45 PM

Anonymous said...
hi, erica! i have been thinking about you each and every moment, and i am
so happy to read that you're heading home - that's fantastic. i thought i'd
posted a comment earlier, but i can't find it above, so i'll just say again that
you're so strong, and courageous, and inspiring....

i am sending you prayers and love, and look forward to meeting you when
you come to boston to visit kendra...

thank you for reminding us all what's important in life...

caroline
January 23, 2011 9:06 PM

Yumi said...
Thanks for the updates! Our prayers, hearts, & thoughts are with you!
You're awesome and we love you!
January 23, 2011 10:02 PM

Anonymous said...
Thinking of you tonight and praying that tomorrow is the day to say
goodbye to that pesky birthmark you have lived with for far too long.
Praying that they will clearly know just what to do.

xo deb (coco's friend in redmond)
January 23, 2011 10:10 PM

Anonymous said...
Sending you more love than you'll know what to do with and hopefully
enough prayers to get all the desires of tomorrow's test. I love you and I
have great faith that whatever the outcome tomorrow, you have made it
to the top of Mt. Everest and after tomorrow, you can put your flag in the
ground and proudly walk down, knowing that YOU have done all that
YOU can do in this journey at this exact point. i love you. Coco
January 23, 2011 10:22 PM

Tanya said...
Dear Erica,

Thinking about you today!

~John and Tanya
January 24, 2011 9:41 AM

Anonymous said...
Erica

I am thinking about you today, and keep hitting refresh on your blog,
hoping for the update! So nice to be able to check in on what is going on.
Thinking about you!!

xoxo
Miranda
January 24, 2011 11:30 AM


On Sun, Jan 23, 2011 at 8:47 PM, Karl Egge wrote:

If sensory and operable we learned she might say no. Lot of sensory
feelings (not able to recognize the shape of coffee drink in car, dig for keys
in pocket without looking) we don't think much about. Bottom line is
there is a "cost" to taking out the birthmark. She is quite reluctant,.I would
do it, but I was told by Becky I can't tell her what I would do!

From: Kendra
Date: Sun, Jan 23, 2011 at 8:48 PM
Subject: Re: Last thoughts over Greek dinner
To: Karl Egge

I agree with Becky... seeing as she will be the one to live with the results!
I hope the decision/tradeoffs become more clear tomorrow... (and I really
hope the "cost" appears lower tomorrow). Hope you enjoyed the Greek
dinner and get some sleep tonight.

Date: Sun, 23 Jan 2011 8:55pm
Subject: Surprise visit? From: Eve

Hi Becky-

I know tomorrow is a huge day and I'm so glad that this limbo period is

112

almost over. It was so good to Skype with Erica today:-).

My husband (very sweetly) wants to buy me a plane ticket to come out and see Erica.....possibly next weekend. Before I even look at tickets, I'm wondering if that's something that is okay with you? I know there's a chance that she might still be in Rochester (although it sounds like based on the timeline you gave last night that maybe she'll be back up in St. Paul by then?), but I'd be happy to stay at that hotel close by if so. If she is home, I could also stay at a hotel so as not to impose on you and Karl when she's home and newly recovering-totally up to you. I want to spend time with Er, be able to help out with her care (maybe give you and Karl a chance to take care of yourselves!), and just generally hold her hand. It looks like the airport isn't too far from your house, so I assume taking a cab or renting a car would be easy enough.

If this is the wrong time I absolutely understand! I just thought I'd ask, because I don't think I'd be able to get out there until March if it isn't this weekend. Either way, please don't tell Er as I'd love to surprise her-I'll bring some Denver sunshine with me!

Let me know! Hugs to you and Karl!

Eve

Date: Sun, 23 Jan 2011 9:20pm
Subject: Big day From: Margaret

Becky,

Have been following the latest on the blog.

Great news that Erica was feeling well enough to Skype with friends.

Will be rooting for the best possible outcome on Monday. There's so much love supporting her, it's bound to work out for the best.

Love to you, deep breath and I hope you are getting a good night's sleep tonight.

Aunt Margaret

On Mon, Jan 24, 2011 at 9:30 AM, Karl Egge wrote:

Becky and I were asked about 8:30 or so to go to the waiting room as the neurologist (Dr. W. - with MD/PHD!) with voltage equipment and staff wanted to do the testing on Erica in her ICU room w/o us around. He said 30% or so chance she could have a seizure induced by the voltage in the test, in which case they had the drugs all set to go ... but, would have to abort the test for the time being ... just didn't want more folks around than necessary. So, add that "RISK" to all the others.

By the way, he said the area where seizures comes from is roughly 1 inch by 1 inch.

We are understanding we could be in this waiting room perhaps 2 hours. Then, my understanding is, we get called back to her ICU room where she is and he talks about the test results, implications, consequences, options, etc.

Assuming no seizure in the test (above) sometime later she goes back to surgery to put the skull back on without or with a surgical step on the 1 inch spot. At that time we again go back to the waiting room.

It was not until last night that I "got it" that if it sensory and not motor, then they can resect (i.e, operate), BUT there is a price to be paid. It is not as simple as taking off a mole or wart. The resection's price is you will lose some sensation. The tests right now are trying to determine where and by how much. The discussion following the tests involves trying to get handle on how high the price she is willing to pay... for good chance to give up seizures how much willing to endure the other way (e.g., maybe can't sense your hand reaching for something in the back seat while you are driving - instead you have to use your head and eyes to watch (ie. guide) your hand to do all these tasks.

I am rambling. We are scared. Becky is reading her rosary!

Love ya all

Karl

Date: Mon 24 Jan 2011 9:58am
Subject: The stimulation mapping is underway From: Mom

Erica is on cruise control. She is worried a) that the stimulation will cause a seizure, 30 to 40 per cent chance; or 2) that there will not be a clear answer as to the advisability of resection and she will be faced with a tough decision. Since all of these uncertainties are out of her control, we just said a prayer that her team be focused and inspired, that the test goes smoothly and leads to a clear answer and that if a decision has to be made God give her the guidance and strength to be at peace that she has made the best decision for herself. If she has a seizure the timing of all this will be up in the air because they will not be able to finish the mapping. As to the decision, Erica does not want to have to decide to trade one deficit for another. We hope the doctors can make a recommendation. She/we have a lot of confidence in them. So pretty tense next couple of hours.

Subject: RE: The stimulation mapping is underway From: Aunt Valerie

Ok. I'm praying with you. Love, Valerie

Subject: RE: The stimulation mapping is underway From: Aunt Martha

Thanks for the update. I am also praying this morning. Please keep me posted.

Subject: RE: The stimulation mapping is underway From: Coco

I've been praying all of those things since I talked to you last night, and once again this morning when I saw the clock at 6am. Sending lots of love, C

Subject: RE: The stimulation mapping is underway From: Eve

We're praying for you....

Subject: RE: The stimulation mapping is underway From: Greta

> anything new? i feel so helpless.
> love
> Greta

Subject: RE: The stimulation mapping is underway From: Mom

I miss you. Erica made it through the test without a tonic-clonic (grand mal) seizure. Whew! Now she needs to decide if she is willing to accept a likely sensory problem with her right hand. Send me a joke or a prayer.

Subject: RE: The stimulation mapping is underway From: Greta

oh my gosh i am sooooo happy!!! I feel bad for being so doubtful but I have been praying this morning and last night too.

This is wonderful wonderful news. I wish I could be with you and feel a little sense of relief. I would make you pause from your rosary to read a little of that sex column from Esquire. I bet you need a laugh after this long stretch of anxiety, waiting, praying, hoping, etc.

I miss you very very much.
love,
g

Subject: RE: The stimulation mapping is underway From: Mom

The test is over and she made it without a seizure. The motor part will be safe but the sensory part will be affected to some extent. Mostly the sense of where her hand is. The doctor described it as a moderate impairment and said her brain would learn to accommodate it to some extent so it would be less of a problem over time Erica is weighing her options and looking forward to talking to the surgeon.

Sent from my iPhone

Subject: RE: The stimulation mapping is underway From: Coco

PRAISE the Lord! So, when I was praying this Bible quote came to me. "For I know the plans I have for you," declares the LORD, "plans to prosper you and not to harm you, plans to give you hope and a future." Jeremiah 29:11

Then I was thinking about how I've heard and seen this over and over before, but maybe you guys haven't. It's called Father's Love Letter - essentially, a compilation of a bunch of Bible quotes that just show you how much God loves you. So with the risk of sounding overly religious, I want to share these with you. Think of them in terms of you, but also in

116

terms of how much God loves Erica, your little baby, more than you'll ever humanly be able to:

Father's Love Letter

My Child ~

You may not know me, but I know everything about you ~ Psalm 139:1 I know when you sit down and when you rise up ~ Psalm 139:2 I am familiar with all your ways ~ Psalm 139:3 Even the very hairs on your head are numbered ~ Matthew 10:29-31 For you were made in my image ~ Genesis 1:27 In me you live and move and have your being ~ Acts 17:28 For you are my offspring ~ Acts 17:28 I knew you even before you were conceived ~ Jeremiah 1:4-5 I chose you when I planned creation ~ Ephesians 1:11-12 You were not a mistake, for all your days are written in my book ~ Psalm 139:15-16 I determined the exact time of your birth and where you would live ~ Acts 17:26

You are fearfully and wonderfully made ~ Psalm 139:14 I knit you together in your mother's womb ~ Psalm 139:13 And brought you forth on the day you were born ~ Psalm 71:6 I have been misrepresented by those who don't know me ~ John 8:41-44 I am not distant and angry, but am the complete expression of love ~ 1 John 4:16 And it is my desire to lavish my love on you ~ 1 John 3:1 Simply because you are my child and I am your father ~ 1 John 3:1 I offer you more than your earthly father ever could ~ Matthew 7:11 For I am the perfect father ~ Matthew 5:48 Every good gift that you receive comes from my hand ~ James 1:17 For I am your provider and I meet all your needs ~ Matthew 6:31-33 My plan for your future has always been filled with hope ~ Jeremiah 29:11 Because I love you with an everlasting love ~ Jeremiah 31:3 My thoughts toward you are countless as the sand on the seashore ~ Psalm 139:17-18

And I rejoice over you with singing ~ Zephaniah 3:17 I will never stop doing good to you ~ Jeremiah 32:40 For you are my treasured possession ~ Exodus 19:5 I desire to establish you with all my heart and all my soul ~ Jeremiah 32:41

And I want to show you great and marvelous things ~ Jeremiah 33:3 If you seek me with all your heart, you will find me ~ Deuteronomy 4:29 Delight in me and I will give you the desires of your heart ~ Psalm 37:4 For it is I who gave you those desires ~ Philippians 2:13 I am able to do more for

you than you could possibly imagine ~ Ephesians 3:20
For I am your greatest encourager ~ 2 Thessalonians 2:16-17 I am also the
Father who comforts you in all your troubles ~ 2 Corinthians 1:3-4

When you are brokenhearted, I am close to you ~ Psalm 34:18 As a
shepherd carries a lamb, I have carried you close to my heart ~ Isaiah
40:11

One day I will wipe away every tear from your eyes ~ Revelation 21:3-4
And I'll take away all the pain you have suffered on this earth ~ Revelation
21:3-4

I am your Father, and I love you even as I love my son, Jesus ~ John 17:23
For in Jesus, my love for you is revealed ~ John 17:26 He is the exact
representation of my being ~ Hebrews 1:3 He came to demonstrate that I
am for you, not against you ~ Romans 8:31 And to tell you that I am not
counting your sins ~ 2 Corinthians 5:18-19 Jesus died so that you and I
could be reconciled ~ 2 Corinthians 5:18-19 His death was the ultimate
expression of my love for you ~ 1 John 4:10 I gave up everything I loved
that I might gain your love ~ Romans 8:31-32 If you receive the gift of
my son Jesus, you receive me ~ 1 John 2:23 And nothing will ever separate
you from my love again ~ Romans 8:38-39 Come home and I'll throw the
biggest party heaven has ever seen ~ Luke 15:7 I have always been Father,
and will always be Father ~ Ephesians 3:14-15 My question is ~ Will you
be my child? ~ John 1:12-13 I am waiting for you ~ Luke 15:11-32 Love,

Your Father

From: Karl Egge
Date: Mon, Jan 24, 2011 at 10:22 AM
Subject: Good news!
To: Kendra, Coco, Greta, Eve, Paul, Martha, Marian, Gladys, Pete, Jessica

We just got called in by Dr. W. She had no seizure. The affected area is not
motor. Part of it is primary sensory (specifically the hand's sensation), but
most of it is secondary sensory (e.g., she would say "weird feeling, but not
sure what it is" and nothing showed up). So, odds are quite high she will
have resection.

Next is to see Dr. M, the surgeon. Hopefully he finishes his AM duties,
gets up here, gives a "go" and the operation is this afternoon.

There are risks, but they are fewer.

I cried and Erica smiled

Love dad/Karl


## BSU #6: Cautiously Optimistic

Just in from Karl and Becky:

The test is over and she made it without a seizure. The motor part will be safe but the sensory part will be affected to some extent. Mostly the sense of where her hand is. The doctor described it as a moderate impairment and said her brain would learn to accommodate it to some extent so it would be less of a problem over time.

Erica is weighing her options and looking forward to talking to the surgeon....although Karl things that the odds are high that she'll go ahead with the resection.

Erica-You are a ROCKSTAR of the highest order!!!! Go Erica Go!!!!!


## Battleship Tongue
(As dictated to my dad)

The circuit board looks like a game of Battleship. "36-37," the doctors called to each other as they stimulated the electrodes in my head one by one. Press one button and my hand would jerk, one my lip would twitch, one my tongue would stick to the roof of my mouth. I couldn't see it, because it was all behind my head. But when I commented on how it reminded me of the game I played as a child, the doctor laughed and said "looking for the motor strip is indeed like looking for the battleship."

Two hours later, the doctor called my parents back from the waiting room and referenced the by now multi-colored pen drawing of the grids on my brain showing where they found the motor strip. Surgery is hopefully scheduled for later this afternoon. And now what is left is to make the decision: To resect, or not to resect. I am obviously waiting to see what the surgeon says, but these are the best results we could have hoped for.

People around the globe have been praying and I thank them all for this is indeed good. There are, however, prices – as there are for anything good. If I complete the resection there is a chance I will lose some of the sensory functions in my right hand. Then again, didn't I know there were going to be prices? Clearly there are, because I have three big grids in my brain and a head wrap that says "No Bone Flap Left Side."

I have to pause to press my pain button, and hear the beep behind me.

I cannot begin to describe how wonderful everyone here has been - the nurses, the doctors, the techs, and everyone with me in my heart. And, Dr. Jack the Helping Dog, who joined our family from the Mayo gift store on Thursday. I have been surrounded by caring thoughts and prayers, family who came when I had a washcloth over my eyes because the light was too bright, and nurses who periodically have to milk my catheter. Despite all this support I am looking forward to going home. No, it will not be for a few days, but after the 2nd surgery I will be able to focus on healing completely versus the partially healed limbo that I have hung in the past 4 days.

I haven't yet seen my half-shaven head, but I am anxious to do so. Anxiously anxious. Last night I ate my first meal since coming here and can't wait to have another. There's gunk under my fingernails and in my ears and there is an awful kink in the left side of my neck where I have not been able to turn since my brain hole lies on that side. There is scum on my teeth and my face is greasy, especially at the border under my bandage. I am quite the sight! I am sure I have acquired many new zits, but hopefully the brightest feature is my smile at the news I received.

## Signing The Second Consent Form

"So, do you want to go through with the resection?" the surgeon asked after doing his best to graphically illustrate the speechless, one-armed life I would surely lead if I said yes.

I thought to myself, Everything has gone perfectly so far, there's no way it's not gonna work. I looked briefly to my parents, gaging their reactions though my mind was already made up. "Yeah, I'll do it."
The nurse slid the consent form onto the hospital table that spanned the width of my bed and still held the lunch I had no intention of touching.

I looked at the little black letters, noticing how they contrasted with the white paper, and how that hurt my eyes. I figured it was the same form I'd signed last time, back when reading didn't give me a headache, so when the pen dropped onto the plastic tray, the bottom rolling in a wide arc as the tip stayed pointed toward the center, I picked it up and scrawled an illegible signature on the open line that I assumed was for such life-altering signatures given while hopped up on hospital-approved narcotics. The paper was whisked away in the same sudden wind that carried the doctors out of my room, presumably before I could change my mind. The ICU nurse babysitting me watched me with a look that I hoped was awe at my courage rather than awe at my wanton stupidity. I could see my parents give each other a deep breath, okay, then, look, steadying themselves before squeezing my hands and smiling at me.

A small part of me asked, What the hell did you just do?, but it was quickly answered, What the hell else was I doing here? Duh. This was exactly what I'd come here to do: get my life back. I was here, lying in bed, too weak to sit up or feed myself, full of pain killers that made me nauseous and fuzzy but that still couldn't take away the pain so strong it made my thoughts hurt, and scared out of my mind because I wanted to try; I needed to try. This was my chance to do what it might take, however extreme, to get a new lease on life. Maybe my chance of success was low, certainly a hell of a lot lower than I'd thought when I started this three months ago, but there was a chance. Prayer, luck, support and courage had gotten me this far, had protected me from every wrong turn I could've taken, and now I was given the choice to have a surgery that could change my life. Yes, there were maybe's, there were prices, but there was so much love holding me up that I knew I could do it, I knew that of course it would work, I knew that my surgeons wouldn't be navigating on their own.

Over the past weeks, I had received so many cards, so many letters (electronic and handwritten), so many calls, all wishing me the best, all sure that everything would be just fine. But even more, everyone said they were praying for me. Family said they were going to prayer group that night; friends of friends whom I'd never met said their church choir was praying for me, adding that "when the prayers go up, the blessings rain down." I was overwhelmed when I heard their stories. My eyes filled with tears more than once and my heart overflowed with gratitude like a beautiful fountain with coins covering its drain.

Of course it was gonna work; there was too much love for it not to.


On Mon, Jan 24, 2011 at 11:21 AM, Karl Egge wrote:

Dr. M came by. Surgery today (they will take her down we think about 1 or 2PM CST), and she decided she will have him do the resection prior to bone stuck back in. So far she has made it through all the negative probability options - it is a miracle so far and it is due in large part I have to believe to so many people praying and hoping for her.

Now the remaining probabilities out of this last meeting:

* 10-15% chance following surgery she will have facial numbness and/or some speech/recall issues (Dr. W had not mentioned that - he only mentioned the hand issue)

* 55-60% chance of seizure free (w/meds still), but Dr. W had said 70% She is riding a hot hand so far and just keep praying and hoping for a few more good things to go her way!

Love ya all

Dad/Karl
On Mon, Jan 24, 2011 at 11:54 AM, Mary wrote:

 Karl, great to hear your enthusiastic good report. Sounds like Grandma Marie is up there pulling some strings.

I am thrilled with the progressive good news. This has got to be a real test of being powerless. I can't imagine how hard it is. I am still praying for all of you. I am home from AZ and hope to make it down to Rochester sometime this week. Love to all of you and a big hug along with it.

Mary

From: Karl Egge

To: Kendra, Coco, Greta
Sent: Monday, January 24, 2011 2:40:05 PM
Subject: no more news at 1:37PM CST

Becky and I just sitting beside her. She is asleep. Obviously they have not come to get her to take her to surgery so far.

Becky and I are both a bit overwhelmed and sort of fragile. This is a big very big thing she got herself into, and there sure appears to be some good light ahead!
More later!

Love dad

From: Greta
Date: Mon, Jan 24, 2011 at 2:44 PM
Subject: Re: no more news at 1:37PM CST
To: Karl Egge

I am praying, hoping, crying and loving you all.
g


## Rolled Into The Second Surgery

The OR was booked for me. The surgeon told me so. So did my nurse, but here I was, still in my room, getting antsier by the minute. Machines whirred behind me, brain juice drained into the plastic bag behind my shoulder and the bandage on my hand where the old IV had been taken out earlier itched. After so many days, the IV port had gone bad - dried up, stale, I don't know - and had hurt, so they moved it over to the other hand. The IV for my anesthetic would be placed after I was tucked in by a plastic gas mask. Somehow the room seemed more tense than before my first surgery. I wasn't sure why and didn't want to guess.

Not until about 2pm did the nurse finally get the call to bring me down to the surgical floor. I said goodbye to my parents as they each squeezed a hand, not wanting to let go. They kissed me on the cheek and said they love me, and just like that I was gone.
My memories of that day have faded into a mist of anesthesia and blocked out fear and pain. They come back to me in vignettes, curtains pulled back to reveal a short snippet of a scene before closing again, hiding the rest from my view. Protecting me.

The elevator door dinged and slid open to reveal an overweight cleaning lady with a rolling cart of mops and antiseptic fluids. She gave us a look tinged with anxiety, not sure if she should leave or stay. I said, "It's fine!" The nurse echoed, "There's room," as she rolled me in, maneuvering expertly around the obstacle. The cleaning lady watched me, wondering if it was rude or voyeuristic of her to be there with me, briefly entering my world in such an intimate and reflective moment. I smiled at her, "Hi! How are you?"

I could see her body relax and she gave an almost laughing smile back, "Good, how are you?"

"I'm fine, thanks. About to have brain surgery again!"

The nurse guided me off of the elevator and down a hallway where we had to pull over and wait for what felt like an hour but was probably only ten minutes until we could enter the pre-op/recovery room. This time I became nervous. My EEG tech new friend, Sydney, wasn't there. She wouldn't be in my surgery today. I looked around, watching doctors, nurses and techs rush past me, this way and that, glancing or not glancing at me on their way. I was alone; empty and full at the same time. I wanted to be brave, but I was scared. Terrified. I reminded myself that I wanted to get the grid out, that it had become very uncomfortable, the way I imagine a pregnant woman is two weeks before giving birth: I wanted it out of me.

The scene fades and suddenly I'm in the operating room. On my back, bright lights pointed at me, it seemed that the whole room was crowded around my head, staring at me, waiting for something. A man came forward through the wall of people and looked at me kindly, sympathetically. Though I could only see his eyes between his surgical mask and scrub cap, I knew he was smiling. "I told Sydney I'd look out for you," he said, taking my outstretched hand in his. Someone took my other hand and I felt more people touching my arms, legs, shoulders. I felt their warmth, their support, as the plastic gas mask was lifted onto my face. "Just breathe, you're gonna be fine. You're doing great," the man said, and I believed him. Then everything went black.

**Surgery 2 Update #1**

She rolled into the OR at approximately 2:45 CST. Karl guesses they won't have any news until about 6 or 7 PM. I'm glad Erica is able to 'sleep' through all of this. We're all nervous enough for her as it is!!

The stats from Dr. M this afternoon:

* 10-15% chance following surgery she will have facial numbness and/or some speech/recall issues

* 55-60% chance of seizure free (with continued medication)

Seizures, you've given Erica almost 20 years of frustration and anxiety. I'm not sorry to see you (hopefully permanently!!) gone. Erica's got bigger and better things to worry about! Adios, birthmark!

3 comments:

Chris said...
Go Erica!!!!!

We're with you! A couple more hours and hopefully you'll be through!

Good vibes to you, your family, and your amazing medical team!
January 24, 2011 3:03 PM

Anonymous said...
Dear Erica, I am so proud of you for being so incredibly STRONG!!! You are amazing! Keep hanging in there- its almost over! Wishing and praying for the best possible outcomes. It sounds like the benefits of being seizure-free far out-weigh the risks of sensory difficulties. And as mentioned in the previous posts, those can improve with time & physical/occupational therapy. It sounds like you & your family have made a well-informed decision, and I am so glad the 'birthmark' is able to be removed! I'm thinking of you & sending a virtual >HUG!< to you & your parents! Love, Natalie
January 24, 2011 5:14 PM

Susan said...
So...I forgot my phone when I went out this morning and couldn't check the blog. Grrrr. Eve called Miff to say Erica was in her 2nd surgery and they were closing her up @ 4:10 PST. Phew!

Erica, welcome to what we all pray is a seizure-free life. A stop by the

PT station, then on to getting on with your new life. We are so hopeful and giddy with all we've heard. We send our best wishes to you and your wonderful family and thanks to the medical team who have treated you with respect, expertise, humor and caring. Most of all, we honor you for your bravery "under fire". We are in awe of your courage and intelligence. Tonight we will raise a glass of wine to toast you as you face your future and all it holds.

All our love,
Susan and Miff
January 24, 2011 6:11 PM


**Surgery Number 2 is Done**
8pm, Just in from Becky:

Surgery is done and Dr. M said it went well. He mentioned that 2 blood vessels went through the part he removed and he was able to work around them. When she is totally closed up (by the resident), Dr. M will check on her in the recovery room, where she has to be for about an hour. Then she is brought back up to the ICU room where she has been. Takes 20 minutes to get her all rehooked up to monitors, minus the grid, and we finally get to see her! She will be in the ICU for a day. Then to the 9th floor rehab. So --- big day. Another one tomorrow when we see how she is awake.

I pray that the worst is over, and that from now on Erica is recovering, recovering, recovering and nothing else! I'll sleep well tonight knowing that the surgeries are done.


**My Worst Memory**

From the sweet depths of anesthesia, my mind began to come back to me. Darkness faded to bright, stark, harsh light and then it hit me. The pain was like nothing I had ever experienced and I hope to God I never do again.

I heard the sound of hysterical sobbing before I realized it was me. The fog around me was disappearing and I so badly wanted it back. People came over to me, though I couldn't say if they rushed or meandered, jaded to the horror. My body writhed beneath me like a snake with a stake driven

126

through it, pinned to the earth. I still hadn't opened my eyes; the filtered light inside my eyelids was already too bright. Then there were voices, ordering me to speak, to open my eyes, let them know I was awake and doing alright. I was not alright. This was nothing, nothing, like the surgery before it, whose gradual end brought a slow awakening that I don't even remember. No, this was not right. Something was wrong.

I opened my eyes only a slit and screamed, snapping them shut with the force of a slammed door.
"Can you tell us what your pain is on a scale of one to ten?" they coaxed.

Sobs wracked me as I all but shouted, "Twelve! Twelve! Please help me! Please! Help me! Make this stop! Make it stop!" I didn't know what I'd done to deserve this. My head would've hurt less if it was still sliced open. My arms moved, my legs moved, my torso thrashed up and down, anything at all that might possibly make it better.

"Okay, you have to calm down. We're giving you pain meds now." I couldn't tell if the woman was exasperated or frightened. Maybe she was both.

"It's not enough! It's not enough! I need more! Help me, please!!" I cried. I couldn't believe that pain like this existed. I couldn't believe that someone would ever let you feel it.

"You need to calm down," she said authoritatively, her voice, as far as I could tell, devoid of concern or sympathy. "You're going to be okay. We can't give you any more pain meds right now."

"No! You have to! You have to!" I couldn't bear it. I couldn't. No. No. I couldn't.

She hesitated momentarily and I can picture her giving a concerned look to her colleague, silently asking if she could. "Okay, I'm gonna see what I can do."

"Thank you, thank you, help me," I was too tired to scream and my desperate pleas faded almost to a whisper, my sobs a terrified, anguished, helpless whimper. Tears cascaded from my eyes like a vicious waterfall, threatening to never stop as long as the world turns. My body was too tired to continue its violent struggle against the pain inside of it and I collapsed inward, limp. The pain was astounding and I wondered how it could ever cease.

There my memory goes black.

## Telling Mom

It wasn't until the next day that I told my parents. I knew how scared they'd already been, the strength they'd mustered from thin air and each other to make it through the last week, and it wasn't over yet.

My mom held my hand and brushed the greasy, clumped hair from my face. I hesitated; she saw. "What's going on, honey?" she asked.

Should I tell her? She doesn't need to be worried. She deserves to know. I took a breath, "When I woke up from surgery, it was really awful. It hurt a lot. A lot more than the first one. I couldn't stop crying." I recounted as much of the terrible thing as I thought she could handle. Her eyes grew wide, and I'm sure watered though I don't remember, and she stroked my hand, calming the tears that had come back to my own eyes.

"We'll ask the doctor. That doesn't sound right. That doesn't sound right at all. I wonder if somebody messed up."

I didn't want her to bother the doctors cause I didn't want to cause any problems, but I knew she wouldn't have backed down and, honestly, I wanted to know, too. I wanted an answer. I wanted to know what happened.

It wasn't until later that day that the surgeon came in to check on me. I was half asleep, as usual, but my ears perked up when my mom began. I felt a guilty blush force its way into my cheeks as she told him what happened and that it was markedly different from the first surgery and asked him what had happened. I imagine him confidently hesitating, though I don't remember, but I do remember what he said. He explained to us that they can't give pain meds right away because they need to make sure the patient wakes up and is physically okay first.
The answer clearly did not satisfy my mom, but she let him go with an, "okay. It just seemed very off." He apologized but reasserted that it was standard procedure. If that's the case, then standard procedure was not

128

followed after my first surgery. Unless I blocked it out, that is, but I've tried to block this out and I can't.


Date: Tues, 25 Jan 2011 10:08am
> Subject: They want her to go to rehab From: Karl

Moving out of the ICU to rehab was harder than a reformer workout. She has a lot of pain but that is to be expected. When you see the photos during surgery you will see why. The high point was a bowl of fruity pebbles - her first food in over 24 hours. I asked Erica if she had a comment for me to pass on but she is too spent.

Subject: RE: They want her to go to rehab From: Eve

Thank you so much for the updates. How are you holding up? All of my love to her-all of her Pilates workouts have prepared her for this moment! I'll update the blog at my lunch hour.

Subject: RE: They want her to go to rehab From: Coco

Poor dear! It's like living hell, I'm sure! The wonderful thing about the human experience is that time lessens the memory of pain's intensity - so yes she'll look back and remember that it hurt like hell, but she won't FEEL that pain when remembering. Ah, the balm of time! Bet you wish some would pass to get her to that heavenly place!


**Post Surgery: Day 1**

Hooray for being done with the surgeries! First and foremost: Erica is doing really well. They have moved her out of the ICU (hooray!) and down to the 9th floor, which is a rehab floor. So far she has no speech delays or major issues with her right hand-what an incredible blessing!

I very happily got to speak to her during lunchtime, and it was great to hear her voice. She is exhausted and in a lot of pain, but (as always) remains positive and thrilled to be on this side of the surgeries. She has a half-shaven head, where you can see the large section of her head that was stapled back, and a drain tube that is draining out blood and 'brain juice' (Karl's words!).

I haven't heard the details from the doctors yet, but I think her moving from the ICU to the rehab floor and her ability to talk is clearly a sign of surgery success! When I get another update on what the doctors have said, I promise to pass it along.

Some of you have asked about sending cards/letters to Erica. The hope is that she won't be in the hospital for too long, so if you send them to her house in St. Paul she'll certainly get them. Although she is exhausted, she asked me to tell you how amazed she is at the outpouring of love from each and every one of you. It doesn't surprise me since Erica has so many people who she has loved and been there for, but it is astounding how many are cheering her on from far and wide, and even those of you who haven't met her. Thank you for joining Team Erica!

4 comments:

Gerry said...
I'm Glad to hear that things went well and that she is on her way to recovering!
January 25, 2011 1:55 PM
Chris said...
Erica,

Great to hear you're out, your head is in one piece, and you've got the same inspiring attitude!

Keep the updates coming
January 25, 2011 9:09 PM

Jim said...
Erica,

So glad you are out of the second surgery and feeling well. Stay strong! Team Erica rocks!

Jim
January 25, 2011 10:52 PM

**Recovery: Day 2**
From Karl this morning:

Erica has been asleep most of the morning. Her right eye is nearly swollen closed. When she is awake it takes awhile for her to form and get out words (nurse said that is the narcotics). I noticed this when talking to her on the phone, too. I cannot begin to imagine what a 'brainstorm' she's been through - so this makes absolute sense. While they want her to rehab, she is in no hurry. Karl says they are hoping to get her out of bed and into a chair to practice sitting. In the ICU she had a one-on-one nurse, and on the rehab floor the nurse has many patients so it's been hard for her to make a whole lot of gains without the help.

Becky headed to the Cities a bit ago not returning until late tomorrow night.

Erica now has a pain patch on her back. Its purpose is to help with headaches. She's been taken off the Percocet, but still has her self-administered PCA which gives oxycodone for pain. They would like to work her down (necessary for going home), but the nurse says you want to stay in front of the pain - so true.

We originally had an estimate of when she might be going home, but it is sounding like it might take longer than expected (Friday? Saturday even?) with how she's feeling. Thank you for the prayers to help her feel better - she needs them.


**2nd day Post Surgery #2 .... On the Recovery**

Erica had a good day. She had her catheter removed. She had her PCA removed. She had her IV removed. So, she is not hooked into or wired into anything. She used a walker to get to the bathroom. She is not in much pain. She is tired a lot. And, she has some nausea, which they are treating.

Dr. S. (neurologist) came by about 3:30 PM and said medically no reason she has to remain here, so he said target leaving for home tomorrow (Friday) – but be flexible based on her condition.
Aunt Martha was down most of the day and helped out (a lot – gave me a reprieve). Becky had to go today to the Cities for a conference, but coming back early this evening.

A wild berry smoothie from Caribou this morning, which she finished over about 3 hours, was the best food intake. Breakfast was highly anticipated, but after a short go at it, she gave it and the pills up (yes, you understand!) Lunch went better, but with a delay. Sort of amusing if you are the dad egging on Egge: Lunch came about 12:30, she wanted to sleep so I asked/said ½ hour until 1PM (OK), wake her at 1 and she wants to sleep more saying I am too bossy, so I say 15 minutes more of sleep (OK) and then eat, so I wake her 1:20 and she isn't happy, so 10 more minutes (OK), and finally gets up out of bed and into a chair. (I was a liberal, right?) She ate perhaps ¼ of her salad and spaghetti. Then she was bit nauseated and wanted to hit the rack again.

I have looked back on the many emails to me over the past week from so many people all wishing her well, and the two most frequently used expressions (which I want to use going forward with you all when you or yours need it) are, "we are sending you good vibes" and "we are praying for you." Well, both of those have worked miracles for Erica. We are so thrilled that she passed all the screens, that both surgeries went well, and that the torture and fear of the last week are in the rear view mirror. We are overwhelmed and humbled and grateful to how many of you have endured along with us this tough saga. Makes me want to shed a tear on all our behalves. I think I will!

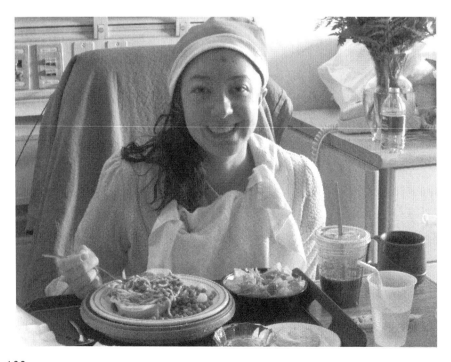

## Going Home Friday the 28th

Becky and I are going to take Erica to St. Paul today. She still is in pain, still needs lot of sleep, but the doctors and nurses are making all the moves associated with "you are out of here today". So, we are packing up her room, have to pack up from our motel room, and then go the pharmacy for her cocktails and then probably to the business office. In some senses it seems premature to go home, but recovery is in stages and not all stages have to be done in a hospital. Thanks for all the support.

Erica says to tell her friends and family she loves them, and she will "post" as soon as she can!

2 comments:

Anonymous said...
Welcome home Erica!! I can't wait to talk to you! It'll be so great to sleep in your own bed:-). Love you, Evie
January 28, 2011 9:43 AM

Anonymous said...
Hi, Erica, Karl, and Becky,
We know it's scary to leave the hospital. However, you are lucky to be so near good medical care in the Twin Cities, also, in case of an emergency.

In the meantime, we're sending you all good vibes for continuous good progress in your recovery! Love, Aunt Gladys & Uncle Laurie
January 28, 2011 10:36 AM


## Cracking my Knuckles

I have an image of someone stretchng their arams long, their fingers wiggling as they streach their head side to side, readying for a race. I like that. In this, my first foray back into typing, I'm not running off the keyboard and diving into the click click rushing water as i breastroke my wy through an ocean of words, picking and chosing from those that float by me. No, my hands are stiff and bruised by five IVs and move clumbsily over the board, leaving me with missed and misspelled words. I can tell that ive lost some sensation and a little control in my right hand, which hopefully will come back soon. I also just took a Percocet, which is bound to make me sleepy and forget words. Fortunately, most words are typed in majority by the left hand. I've also found out that they had to detach my jaw muscle to do the craniotomy, which explains the soreness there.

Well, this has been quite the adventure! Sitting that cold, Rocucester day in the sorgeon's office, when i was told that i have a 25% chance of our little experiment working, I learned something about myself: I'm either inreadibly stubborn and caught a lucky break, or coragous and not alone. I'd like to think the latter, but mayby it's a bit of everything. I've been through hell this week, lying an a recovery table coming off anesthesia and sobbing as i pleaded to the nurses that my pain was a twelve, but today I started to feel my triumph and celebrate my release. Everything that could have gone wrong, every gaping dark tunnel and dead end, let me pass by; a Perfect Storm of Grace.

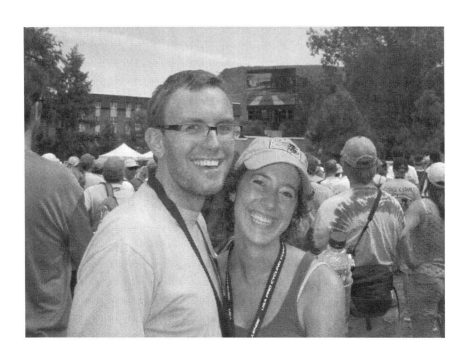

# Part III:
# Recovery

For John: my best friend, my rock,
the love of my life.

## Beautiful Battle Scars

It's Eve again. I am happy to be gradually passing the blogging duties back to Erica(!!), but while she heals and typing is a bit harder for her I am thrilled to help out by updating. I am lucky enough to be in St. Paul with Erica right now-so I can see first hand what an amazing job she is doing healing from such a huge ordeal.

It seems that being released from the hospital helped Erica turn a big corner in her healing process. There's no place like home, and her spirits have been lifted as she relaxes in the comfort of the familiar. She still needs to sleep a fair amount of the day, but when she's awake she is her old self. Correction: She's far better than her old self. She told me she doesn't like how 'ugly' half of her head looks, but I see it so differently.

Though her craniotomy left her with 60+ staples in her head and less-than-perfect use of her right hand, to me it represents the new life she fought so hard to get. In her post yesterday she talked about the luck that went into each phase of these surgeries. Luck was part of it-but I believe that almost 20 years of seizures, doctor appointments, MRIs, side effects, etc. were her payment. She earned this (hopefully!!!) seizure free life, and these beautiful battle scars are the proof of what she had to go through to get it.

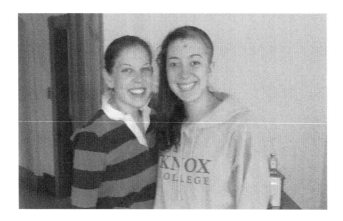

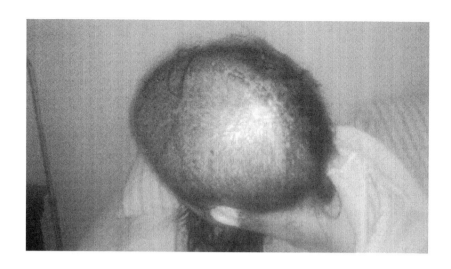

## Scrub-a-Dub-Dub

The water flowed through the pipes in the wall, down the hand-held cord, out the shower head and through my hair. Yesterday, I took my first shower. I sat on a bench, my chin tilted up as my mom rinsed shampoo from my matted hair, carefully cupping the border between locks and peach fuzz to protect the staples. I flashed back to gently cupping the foreheads of my nieces and nephews to keep the suds off their delicate faces as I rinsed shampoo from their fine hair.

I'd kept my green elf hat on since leaving the hospital and as the water ran down, pooling at my feet before making its way to the drain, its red tint betrayed the blood that caused the smell and stiffness of my hair. I pulled handfuls of conditioner through the strands to combat the stench. I used every potion in my store to scrub the hospital from me. I lathered creamy, lavender soap on my arms and brought an elbow to my nose to take in the familiar scent. I shaved my legs with some kind of Ocean Breeze-type gel, focusing on using my right hand and managing not to cut myself, though, admittedly, missing a couple spots.

I called for an assist and closed my eyes as a small trickle of water made its way down my face. The water was losing its heat, and my mom worked quickly to rinse the remaining conditioner from my hair. I pushed in the dial on the tiled wall and the shower head slowed to a drip, drip, and the pipes in the wall quieted.

## So Tired, So Grateful

Yes, I am in pain. I'm exhausted. I'm every facet of overwhelmed. But by far, the dominating emotion is love. Love, and gratitude. It all seems so surreal; the staples and the headaches remind me that it really happened. I'm still processing; I think a lot of us are, and I'm sure we will be for a while.

I'm beginning to write down everything from the hospital before the haze of it melts away into that fog of whirlwind memories. Before I do, though, I have a very special thank you. There's no way to do this properly, no words that could ever express the depth of my gratitude, but in lieu of the right way, I say a humble thank you to my parents. They sat by my bedside, holding my hands and being my rocks, no matter how scared and jumbled they felt inside. They gave countless updates to loved ones around the world. They supported my decisions as I went forward, signing consent forms that we all knew could be risky. They fed me when I was too weak to hold a spoon, too tired to bring water to my lips. They held cold cloths to my eyes, adjusting them around my oxygen tube, when there was just too much pain and my eyelids weren't enough to keep out the light. I can't pretend to know how hard this has been for them, but when I needed them to be strong for me, time after time they rose to the occasion.

It's also important to recognize my three beautiful sisters, who always supported me, teased me as sisters should, prayed with me; my aunts, who drove the hour and a half back and forth to Rochester more than once to hold my hand, my parents' hands, and made me laugh even when it hurt; Eve, who sifted through every email, phone call, text, to faithfully keep the blog, and breathed life into me by surprising me all the way from Denver upon my return home; Jill, who updated the United States' Finest around the world; the doctors, techs and nurses at Mayo; and last but absolutely not least, all of you, who have been with me as I've been on this journey, which still continues.

Last night I lay in bed, a cold cloth over my eyes, my mom holding my hands, and I began to cry. Tears streamed down, sobs threatening, and I couldn't make them stop. The picture of worry, assuming it was pain, my mom asked me what was wrong, but all I could say was, "It all went perfectly." She sighed a relieved smile, "I know it did. It was perfect. But why are you crying?" I shuddered a breath, and replied, "I'm just so grateful. And so tired."

February, 2011

## Picking Scabs

Three small, mostly circular, scabs flanked the large one on my forehead. Oblong, or maybe squarish, I couldn't quite tell, a week after marking their territory they had turned yellow. The edges curled up like peeling paint, threatening to chip at the slightest disturbance from a passing hand brushing away strands of hair. What's left of my hair, that is.

This morning I went on my second excursion since coming home from the hospital Friday afternoon, but this time I made it out of the car, donned in puffy coat, boots and scarf, and traversed the packed snow that lined the sidewalk. Holding onto my mom's arm, I managed to make my way into Jamba Juice and order a smoothie before needing the reprieve offered by the small round table near the door. It felt good to get out of the house, despite the weather, and the stimulation of the blender and employee-chosen music overhead didn't assault my ears the way it would have only yesterday. My mom came back to my nook with smoothie and muffin in hand and took the seat across from me. We deliberated on which setting offered less stimulation, weighing the pros and cons of the shop versus the traffic and passers-by outside; given the inhospitable weather, a fair comparison was not possible, so it came up a draw.

As we stood up from our eight-minute outing, my dear mother cautioned me to be careful not to let the yellow, dried, bubbly skin fall into my Caribbean Passion. In the car, the scabs stared at me from the passenger mirror as we pulled from the snowy curb, taunting me and testing my patience. I flipped the mirror up, attempting to subdue my itchy fingers in their gloves, vowing to wait until getting home. The three minute ride was endless and we talked about my staples and peach fuzz and how to get the remaining dried blood flakes out of my hair; none of which were helpful distractions.

A few blocks later, I disembarked and made my way slowly and steadily across the driveway, through the kitchen, up the stairs and to the bathroom. They were still waiting for me. There were symmetrical marks on either side of my head, too, all on the same latitude and tracing the vice that had held my head while my skull was removed like Silence of the Lambs, but, oh, the off-center bindi, placed half-way between my hairline and eyebrows, drove me nuts.

I'd waited for the proper lighting and mirror to be sure that I wasn't removing living-scab that would be more likely to scar, but after close inspection I got the green light. And I picked the scabs. And it was glorious.

## Naps and Pain Pills

These days have been a marathon of eating and sleeping, differentiated from one another by my overall pain level. Yesterday and the day before were both pretty hard, but until about 7:30pm, today hasn't been too bad. I keep a post-it tracking the number of oxycodones I take - one every four hours as needed to complement the Percocets. Today I've only taken two: 7am and 3:30pm. They always say that you need to, "stay ahead of the pain", and I have to remind myself how hard it is to get back on the train once you've derailed. I take four Percocets every day, at 8am, 2pm, 8pm and 2am, and the oxycodone for "breakthrough" pain. My problem is one that I suspect is prevalent among the population that tends more toward lucidity: I think to myself, "I don't really need it that badly, it's fine. I'll just wait for my next Percocet." Of course, that's a bad idea, and I curse myself later when I flinch at the slightest noise or a room lit at any setting above "romantic." I'm working at anticipating myself and remembering that there's no bravery medal to be won here.

Now I just have to remember my naps. I wake up every morning at 8am to take my pills, brush my teeth, and pad down the stairs (with a spotter) to breakfast. After my fruit, toast, oatmeal and tea (I'm building up a real-people appetite!), I have maybe two hours until my first nap of the day. The past couple days, I've worked on my dexterity by knitting as I listen to a Nicholas Sparks audio book. Despite my mom's efforts to make me a knitter like her, my current project is a rectangular scarf that I began two years ago before leaving in a brown, paper yarn store bag. The yarn is dark, spackled purple and fuzzy enough to mask my crooked stitches. The knitting and typing have been good for my hand though, and I've noticed an improvement in its control; it's not perfect, and maybe it never will be, but it's getting better every day.

Nap #1 is at 11am and goes until 1 or 1:30. At this point I might get to see a visitor if one comes by, and then nap #2 is at 4pm. Today I missed my first nap when a friend came by, equally disoriented by pain pills from her own recent foot surgery, and we spent two hours lying in bed watching the first movie I've seen since the surgery - quite an auspicious play-date! I was, however, gently scolded for skipping my nap, and I made up for it in late-afternoon headaches.

Speaking of which, the dull throbbing of the left side of my head is nagging me to sign off and go to sleep!


## Experiments

Next to my bed, two small dishes sit on my nightstand. They're round and ceramic, handmade with a swirl that spirals out from the center, the width of the finger that dug its pattern out of the clay while it turned on its wheel. The glaze is that blue that might be green, but you can never quite tell because it looks different every time.

The dishes are out of place on my nightstand; they should be individually filled with soy sauce and a touch of wasabi, set on the boarder of a bamboo placemat on a nicely staged table, not surrounded by an empty phone charger, half-drunk glasses of water, a small stack of books my eyes can't focus on yet, and a few get well cards. White pills take the place of a fancy dipping sauce: a Percocet in one and an oxycodone in the other.

My first couple nights back from the hospital, we set my 2am Percocet on top of a magazine so I wouldn't have to get up when my phone alarm chimed me awake. We soon decided that putting the pill in a dish was a little more civilized than leaving it lying around on Johnny Depp's face.

The next night, the second dish was added, when I awoke in pain in the middle of the night, far from pill time, and had to stumble my way, one hand holding my head, to the bottle of little, round oxycodones. That was unpleasant, hence the easy-access dish. Everything was going perfectly, until last night. I tried to piece it together, but I had brain surgery last week, so it was a little difficult. Suffice to say, I woke up at 4am and saw that at 2am I had accidentally taken the oxycodone, not the Percocet. I dropped the narcotic in my mouth and propped myself up on my elbow for a long drink of water. The sky is not falling, but my barely-memorized medicine schedule has now been shifted back two hours. While this might appear to be an accident, I can assure you it is an experiment in mental dexterity... yeah...

I haven't listened to music since the surgery. Except for the rare tv show - a new phenomenon in my life - I am able to handle either visual or

144

simple audio, but not both at the same time. That has led me to choose an audio book over the radio or a cd since a single voice talking is much less stimulation for my fragile ears than music. But yesterday, I was struck with an idea: what would happen if I turned on my ipod? A spark lit inside me, a mix of curiosity and mischief, as I scrolled through the playlists, searching for one that wouldn't hurt my ears, and pushed the Power button on the black dock that looked more like a flying saucer than speakers. A song began to play, an upbeat tune with slightly confusing lyrics that always leave me wondering if the singer just won the guy or was just dumped by him. I didn't care, because something within me broke open, and I smiled as I felt a wall crumble inside of me. I would've danced if I wasn't worried about falling over, but my heart danced and I allowed myself a little wiggle as I supported myself with one hand on my dresser and one on the borrowed walker that's sat abandoned since three days after coming home from the hospital.

The spark inside me jumped and awoke the vocal chords that have lain dormant since the doctors' first incision. Without meaning to, I suddenly found myself singing! One line, one beautiful line shot fireworks through me, but then I grabbed my head and gasped. Every joy has its price, but that wasn't going to deter me, and I bargained with myself for every third line. It was worth the extra oxycodone to burst through the sound barrier covering my soul. The smile almost broke my face, splitting it down a fault bordered by my lips. I ran out of breath after three or four lines and sat down on the edge of my bed, head throbbing, as my physical limitations showed themselves, but I knew this was just the first go, and as soon as I have enough strength, I can't wait to try again.

I feel kind of like I'm meeting myself and exploring the world for the first time. Through my new eyes, I see the truths within myself and I see the goodness and oneness of humanity. Everything is new and has been touched with the kindness that has been shown to me. Rose colored glasses wouldn't do the world justice. Each new day amazes me, the way the sun and moon make the snow sparkle in turn while I watch from my window; the patience I'm shown when I walk slowly, talk slowly, pause as I climb the stairs; the support I've been given by everyone who's read this blog.

## Ice Sculptures

I woke up bleary-eyed and checked the clock: 8:20. I sat up in stages, first adding one pillow to the two I slept on, then pushing myself up on my elbow on top of the pillows, next using my arm as a kickstand as I maneuvered my legs out from under the comforter before finally sitting up. I paused before standing, just to make sure I had my balance, and got to my feet. I walked carefully down the hallway, stopping just before the bathroom, and called out, "Dad, are we still going to the ice sculptures?"

Today, I went on my biggest excursion yet: to see the ice sculptures at the Winter Carnival. I sat shotgun, my mom giving up her seat for the brain patient, while I reminded my dad to drive slowly. The bumpy roads hurt my head, but a greater problem was that I hadn't taken my nausea pills...

Dad dropped us off at the carnival entrance and went to find a parking spot. I held my parents' arms for balance (and warmth) as we crossed the threshold at 9:15. This year is the 125th anniversary of the Winter Carnival. The park where's its held in downtown St. Paul was covered with ice sculptures of all make and model. A wishing well, complete with a bucket attached to a clear, glass-like rope crank got second prize for a single block sculpture, though in my opinion it should've gotten first.

We kept walking, and the cold air felt nice on my face and temples. A grey, knitted beret sat cock-eyed on my head, both masking and protecting the exposed scalp healing underneath it, but was mostly covered by the zipped-on hood of my puffy black coat. As we made our way through the winding sidewalk maze, the multi-block sculptures to our left rose up from the ground, shaped like dragons, trees, fire-god temples.

We walked and walked, me still holding each parent by the arm as we made our way through the park and back. Dad had found a parking spot just across the street, and I made sure to ask him what time we left: 9:30am. I made it fifteen minutes!

And then I went home and took a nap!

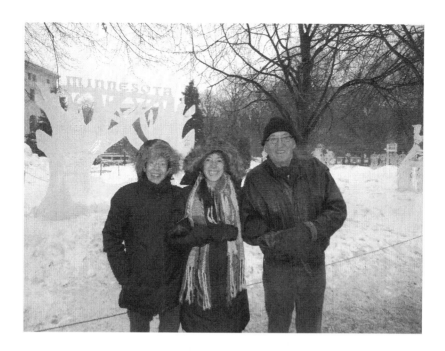

## Weaning

My head hurts. Granted, it's probably got something to do with the fact that there were people playing around in my brain with knives the other week, but it's also in part because I'm turning a corner. At 2am this morning, the dish on my nightstand, blue in the moonlight streaming through my windows and cut by the street lamp on the boulevard two houses down, was filled not with Percocet, but with two extra strength Tylenol. I'm finally starting to wean myself off of the narcotics I've been on since the afternoon of January 20th. As much as the painkillers worked, and I'm grateful for their presence in recent weeks, I can't wait to see them leave. The fogginess, the fatigue, the difficulty remembering words and their orders while speaking, the nausea, the dizziness, I will not miss them. However, my head hurts. Speaking of which, hang on a sec while I grab a barf pill (nausea pill).

The barf pills are fast acting, and are to be disintegrated in your mouth. I put one under my tongue; it tastes like cherry. The fast acting aspect is particularly important since my nausea tends to come on suddenly and be pretty fast acting itself, and I'd rather not have chunks of last night's dinner on my yellow, striped duvet.

Anyway, back to the headache. Since getting home, my regimen has been four Percocets a day: 2am, 8am, 2pm, 8pm, and oxycodone for any breakthrough pain. I would usually end up taking three oxycodones a day. But now, I've replaced the oxycodones with Tylenol. Percocet is actually just Tylenol plus oxycodone, so I have to remember to count those in my daily Tylenol allotment - eight per day. Now, here's my new experiment: replacing two Percocets per day with two Tylenols: 2am and 2pm; 8am and 8pm continue to be Percocets for now. So far, it hasn't been bad. It hasn't been great, but it hasn't been bad. So wish me luck that it works, because I'd like to get on to the next stage!

Ps- I get my head staples out today! I'll let you know how it goes!

**Staples**

I took a deep breath and held on to the banister. The house was empty and I had to go down the stairs. I usually walk them on my own, positioning myself between the banister and the wall, a hand on each, but always with a spotter; never alone and never with no one home. But I had to make it downstairs, I was getting a ride to the family practice physician's to get my staples out. I made sure to wear my fuzzy slippers with the rubber bottoms for extra traction, and took the first step down. Okay. This is okay. I've got this. Next step. Right, left, right, left. I paused at the landing to catch my breath then continued, almost there, almost there, two more stairs, then one. I mercifully touched both feet on the floor and let out an audible sigh of relief. I would have kissed the ground, but bending over makes me dizzy.

No time for breakfast, I ate two lemon bars Eve's mom sent me, the butter and sugar mixing in my mouth and tasting like heaven and love as it made its way to my stomach. Breakfast is by far the best meal of the day, so I made a note to remember it as I put on my Minnesota-chic puffy coat, hat and scarf. I slipped the staple remover given to me when I left Mayo into my purse just as the doorbell rang.

My godfather stomped the snow off his shoes and took them off to come and help me down the last few stairs to the door. I assured him I could make it, but he said, "Nope, you're not falling on my watch." I swapped the fuzzy slippers for proper boots, he re-shoed, bending down to pull the back of each over his heels, and he led me out the door. He held tightly to my arm as he steered me toward the passenger side and lowered me in, pulling the seat belt out and handing it to me.

The clinic was an eight-minute drive at most, and he let me out as he parked against the wall of snow that lined the street. In the waiting room, we made jokes about my brain and the scars on my head until the nurse called us back.

I hung up my jacket and pulled off my boots while the nurse took down the long list of medications I take and asked why I was there: "I have staples in my head and I'd like get them out." She left, the doctor came in, and I again explained that I'd just had brain surgery for my epilepsy and was left with 54 staples in my head and a staple remover as a souvenir. He remembered me from visits long ago and asked about my sister and parents as I hopped onto the exam table. I laid back and, pop!, out came the first staple. It stung, to be sure, but I had been expecting much worse and was pleasantly surprised. My godfather asked where I'd put my phone and how to turn on its camera, and I told the doctor that I needed a picture of this. I don't know if he was amused or annoyed, but he indulged me and paused for me to set up the camera. The doctor proceeded to remove every other staple as my godfather held up the phone, his new mustache hidden behind it, and snapped a picture, the fake camera noise confirming that it'd worked.

Pop, pop, wiggle, pop! Most of the staples came out easily, and I looked forward to scraping the scabs and skin flakes off of the scalp seam once I got home. The doctor paused and announced that a few staples had burrowed their way a bit deeper and would require the use of his forceps. I'm tough, I've been through worse - much worse - it'll be fine, I told myself. And it was. Forceps? Ain't no thang.

Before leaving, the nurse returned and gave me one of those awful finger pricks that hurt more than getting an IV inserted, to test my hemoglobin, which had almost earned me a transfusion before I left the hospital. When I was discharged, it had been at 8.2 versus the 12 where it should be; 8 is when they give you a transfusion. The nurse informed me as I held my throbbing finger, and silently lamented that she hadn't given me a Snoopy Band-Aid, that I'm up to 9.6. Not great, but getting better. I still have to take the iron pills I was prescribed at the hospital for another six weeks, but one extra pill doesn't make too much of a difference in my daily regimen.

Fifteen minutes later, I was home, eating breakfast and picking scabs.

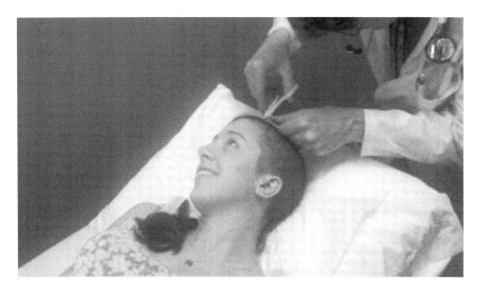

## I Sleep On My Left

I sleep on my left. I like sleeping on my left. I haven't slept on my left for twenty nights. I get into bed, dust a few flakes of head scabs off of my pillowcase, turn off the light, and lie there. On my right. Agonizing.

I roll my head to and fro on the pillow to get the quickly forming cramps out of my neck. I find myself with my chin cocked out and readjust my head backward, in line with my spine, then again readjust my pillow around my face.

My shoulder blade slides out like a dinner plate from under my body, serving up my scrunched shoulder, rotating in its socket as I bring my arm down to my side, up toward my head, somewhere in the middle, whichever feels the least unnatural.

I try to ignore the way that my left side collapses in on me as my body tries to reconcile my torso with the shape of the mattress. My right hip digs into the bed, the poorly-planned fulcrum point upon which all of my weight is not quite balanced.

My knees knock together every time I move, making me contemplate putting a pillow between them to save each from the sharp pound of the other, but though it might also balance my hips, I never actually do so.

The ankles follow suit with the knees, the top one falling off its perch and landing in front, no, behind, no, in front of the other.

Somewhere, a nerve is pinched, and the toes of my right foot spend most of the next day asleep.

Thank goodness I'm so tired!


## Oddities of My New Head

When I push the left side of my skull, I can feel the pressure in my nose.
The forward one third of my scalp is numb.
The back one third is still very tender.


## Two Steps Forward, One Step Back, And Maybe One More Sideways

The headaches are back. Just in the past couple days. The Tylenol was working, and it was so exciting; I was so happy to be off of the narcotics that made me tired, foggy, nauseous, dizzy. But yesterday I took two oxycodoncs for thc pain. It's a dull presence that slowly, ominously, grows. It gets bigger, more pronounced, and a sudden rustling sound or a cough in the next room makes me jump and wince. I just washed my hands and my fingers are cold from the water, so I put them on my face: I cover my cheeks, my forehead, my temples, the back of my neck, turning my hands over after one side loses its cold to the heat of my face. I call for my dad, as quietly as I can while still being effective, and ask him to run downstairs to grab my nausea pills out of my backpack. My body is getting hotter, and I unzip my sweatshirt, taking out one arm and then the other before dropping it on the floor next to me.

The nausea pill tastes like cherries and I hold it under my tongue while it dissolves into my bloodstream, leaving behind a chalky aftermath that I wash away with the glass of ice water waiting on a glass coaster on the coffee table next to me.

My stomach is full of pills. No matter how much I eat, I still feel them, sitting there. So many pills; so many pills. I haven't counted lately how many I take, but it's probably getting up to twenty a day or so. They just sit in my stomach, waiting for something I can't discern. I wish I knew how to wash them away, but all I can do is put another cherry pill under my tongue and hope that this time it'll get better.

That's the hard part, the step back, but I promised good news, progress, too. I feel like I should have a "Baby's First" book to chronicle my accomplishments as I re-introduce myself to normal life. I can now walk up and down stairs by myself, no spotter! I still need someone to carry my things if they weigh more than my mandated maximum ten pounds, or if they present a particularly precarious balancing situation, but otherwise I can fly solo. I can shower without a chaperone, as well. I still sit on a bench as I do so, but I no longer require someone to sit in the bathroom with me to make sure I don't slip and break the eggshell that covers my brain.

My right foot is one of the remnants of my surgery: my toes and the sole of my foot are numb. Not the strong, overpowering numb that they were in the hospital, where I couldn't feel my toes wiggle and pins and needles took turns plaguing me, but it's there, a reminder of what I went through. Sometimes it doesn't feel real, like a faded dream. Even the headaches don't do justice to the tile floors, the cold rooms, the coil that carried the leads through my scalp and into the beeping machines behind me. It's other things that remind me what happened: my numb toes; the pain at the back of my tender head when I turn in my bed to give rest to my right hip; the long curls that cascade, untended, past my right shoulder, that get heavier every day and contrast so strangely with the buzz-cut fuzz that hugs the shape of the left side of my head. It's been growing, though, and yesterday I even started a file of cute short hair cuts that I can hopefully bring to a hairdresser in a matter of two or three weeks. One more remnant disappears.

Yesterday I blow dried my hair for the first time since the surgery. The hairdryer sat on my bathroom sink, just where I'd left it next to the mirror. The diffuser attachment sat maybe four inches away and I held the back of the hairdryer against my stomach as I muscled the purple plastic into place and heard it pop. The air was hot as it coaxed out the curls, and I was careful to protect my peach fuzz, the un-used hand shielding the boarder between shaven and unshaven.

It's progress. It's not easy, it's not quick, and it's not always forward, but it's something. Reentering my life changes every day; a rollercoaster,

152

like so much else, that's mental, physical and emotional. I'm constantly reminded that this is going to take time. I have good days, but I'll pick up a book to find that the words don't stick in my head, and my eyes hurt. Then again, I'll have bad days, but find that screens don't hurt and I can escape into a rerun of an NBC sitcom until I'm able to walk again. The days alternate, but still I add to my repertoire of tricks. I'm more sure of my footing, better able to talk, and make fewer mistakes as I type. It's progress. It's not easy, it's not quick, and it's not always forward, but it's something.


## Twitching Legs

I awoke this morning to a throbbing head. I tried to move, readjust myself and hope it would stop, but each way I turned was worse. I felt nauseous, and it kept throbbing, throbbing; the whole left side. The back of my head was ground zero, the pain radiating away from it, filling the expanse from my ear to the part in my hair as it made its way to and across my forehead. And my jaw, so unceremoniously severed as the surgeons dug their way past my skull, couldn't decide between sharp and dull, so it alternated between the two, keeping rhythm with the beat of my head. My right cheek on the pillow, gravity pulled at my jaw bone and it hung down toward the yellow striped case, tugging at the angry muscle. I tried putting my hand underneath the pillow to prop up my jaw, realigning it with its skull-fused partner, and it sort of worked, for a while, but even so, everything still seemed to hurt. So badly. I thought of the hospital and how I was asked to rank my pain on a scale of one to ten every hour. I estimated myself at a four and remembered the sustained sevens I'd lived for days, interrupted by eights and even nines. And the recovery room after the second surgery... I forced the memory of that night out of my head. Still, I was lucky that I throbbed at a four, that the higher numbers were behind me. That didn't make it stop hurting though.

I dragged myself up, knowing, despite my tired body's protests, that to get to any painkiller I had to stand and walk the three steps to my dresser. I pushed and turned the child protected bottle of oxycodone and washed one down with two Tylenol. I carefully collapsed back into bed, planning to force myself asleep for another half hour until the pills kicked in.

The city is cutting down overhanging branches and dead trees along the boulevard in my neighborhood this week, and the sounds of industrial progress bore a striking resemblance to chainsaws outside my bedroom window. The zip and roar pulled my eyes open over and over, jarring me from sleep no matter how hard I tried. I stared straight ahead at the wall, eyes dry and unfocused, and imagined I looked like a cartoon character, exaggerated bags under bloodshot eyes, a gray pallor to my expressionless face. It didn't help that I didn't sleep well last night.

Everything could be traced back to one thing: my legs. The past few nights - and naps, for that matter - have been poisoned by a twitching in my legs. I lie in bed, 90% asleep, when an energy begins to grow in my legs, reminding me of a defibrillator charging, the paddles rubbing together before shocking my body by the legs, making them jump and twitch almost violently and landing on the bed, daring me to fall back asleep before charging again. Sometimes it helped to switch sides and sleep on my left, but the pain that generated in my head was too much and I turned back over.

Generally, twitchy legs would be at most a potential cause for possible concern, but in my house, any involuntary movement leaves each of us in a state of alarm which we try, unconvincingly, to hide from one another while we pray that it's not a seizure. I can't even begin to convey how hard I pray that it's not a seizure. Ever since I was told that the resection went smoothly, that the short circuit that had plagued my brain and my life was gone, I've walked around on top of the world, assuming that my seizures are gone. I was told as I left the hospital that I have a 70% chance of never having another seizure. Everything had gone so perfectly, more so than we could have hoped, that it never occurred to me I might be in that 30%. Not once; at least not convincingly. At this point I think it might be some form of Restless Leg Syndrome because despite the involuntary convulsion, it doesn't feel like a seizure. Even if it is, I was told that having a seizure sometime in the first few weeks is normal. I'm still wary (and nervous and tired), but I think it's okay. Despite everything, it would take a lot to convince me that I went through that surgery in vain. I'm part of the 70%.

## 134 lbs

I weighed myself today. I don't like to weigh myself. 134. I've gained four pounds since I've been home. That's good, I know, and I'm glad that my appetite has come back and I'm able to keep down all the nutrients that my body needs to heal from its massive ordeal, but old habits die hard. I've been looking at pictures of short hair styles lately, even starting

154

a file on my computer of my favorites that I can print out and bring to the hairdresser in a few weeks. I think about how cute they are and I'm excited to try the kind of hair style that I never would have chanced under different circumstances. So very, very, very short... it'll be fun. But old habits die hard. I think about my new hair and my thoughts immediately go to, "short hair looks better on thin people. You have to be thin to pull it off. I'll have to lose a little weight. Good thing I lost some at the hospital!". No. No, Erica, you cannot just decide to lose weight for a hair cut right after brain surgery. You are not good at losing weight.

I can't stop thinking about it: every time I look at my hair, every time I watch tv, watch a movie, see people on the street. I can't wait to start working out and dieting. Three more weeks before my moratorium on exercise is up. By the time I get back to Denver, I'll be able to get back to Pilates, the gym, zumba once I get adjusted to the altitude, and maybe a dance class, too. I'll be slim and trim in no time and I'll look awesome.

Erica, stop. Breathe. None of those thoughts have a place in your head right now. You just got major, major brain surgery, and you need to recover. Do you want to mess up your recovery? Don't you remember the hell you just went through to get where you are? Don't you? So stop, and breathe, and calm down. Just calm down. You have a job to do right now: get better. That's it, that's your full-time job.

The biggest trigger that causes an anorexic to relapse is a lack of control. When the world is spinning and life is confusing and scary and the answer to every question is, "it depends," there's still one thing you can control. There's a sick comfort in the familiarity of it. No, you can't control life, can't catch every ball thrown in the air, but you can control every calorie, every crumb, that enters your body. When your stomach growls, you can press on, because you're stronger than your body; you have more discipline than that. You dust off your finely tuned logistical skills and remember how to plan your meals and excuses around the people who might notice to keep them in the dark. Even though you know it's wrong, even though you're disgusted with yourself for sliding back into a place you worked so hard to escape from, a twisted glee spreads across your face because you got away with it. You got away with starting again and nobody knows.

I don't like to write these words and I don't like to read them. I don't like that they came from my fingers, and I know that if I word it wrong it could do me more harm than good, but this is a chronicle of my life and this is what's going through my mind. I just have to remember to be strong. Hunger is a toxic feeling, so every time I'm hungry, I will eat. Simple as that. I can do that. I have to do that. I just went through hell and I'll be damned if I mess up all I've gotten for an old ghost.

Eat when I'm hungry. I can do that.

## Debutante

I have officially had my coming out party and have been reintroduced to society as an object for show and tell!

My phone alarm woke me from my nap, G. Love singing to me that "it's about time to get out of bed/ Right about now." He added something about being an astronaut, but as that wasn't really applicable to me, I slid the dismiss button, dropped it on the nightstand and threw back my covers. It was four o'clock, people would be coming in an hour.

My dad had invited some of our neighbors at the cabin to stop by from five to six thirty Saturday evening to see me. He conceded that I was playing the role of dancing monkey for the night, but I was fine with that; I hadn't seen some of the neighbors since summer and I was excited to catch up.

My mom called down to me as I reached the bathroom door to make sure I was awake. I assured her that I was. "Okay," she returned, sounding wary, "Cause they're coming in an hour."

"Okay, mom," I indulged, trying my best to keep the teenager edge out of my voice. I continued to the bathroom and grabbed my toothbrush, applying a layer of toothpaste before remembering I'd meant to bring my computer for some background music while doing my makeup. I shoved the toothbrush in my mouth and began brushing with my right hand as I padded barefoot over the downstairs carpet and scooped my computer off of the nightstand with my left.

Returning to the bathroom, I spat, rinsed, and replaced the toothbrush. I clicked on the 80's station I'd put together on Pandora and adjusted the volume for the smaller, more echo-y room. I so rarely put on makeup these days that it's become a kind of treat. I spend the majority of my time at home not seeing anyone, so it seems silly to bother. But tonight

156

is my cotillion, and I want to look my best. I unscrew and re-screw caps, dabbing and spreading in between; brushes emerge from a rustling bag to lightly apply this powder or that; a rainbow's worth of eyeshadows are spread out and selected from; a small, angular brush with stiff bristles meticulously moves around the edges of my eyes, sweeping and blending to create the dark brown boarder along my lash line; two bristled wands appear side by side and I lean closer to the mirror as I coat my eyelashes first in a white base and then a dark black that threatens to clump even as I watch each lash magically grow. I step back to inspect the full effect: not bad.

I'd laid out my clothes on the bed (read: I knew what I was wearing and it was draped unceremoniously over the top of the gym bag with the broken zipper that sat on my floor), so all that was left was my hair. I tugged out my singular pigtail - when half of your hair is gone, you can't pretend it's still a ponytail - and examined it. The curls were limp, if that, and the bangs that had looked so stylish a month ago formed a wave that betrayed the grease beneath it. I took my hair in one hand and pulled it up and back, holding it for a moment to see what it might look like, but dropped it again to my shoulder. I reached behind my neck to fetch any strays and finger-combed my hair forward before sliding a binder into place below my right ear.

A laundry basket thudded as it hit the ground, and I swung the bathroom door open, "Dad, I need help, how does this look?" I paused but he stared at me blankly. "My hair, dad. How does my hair look? Should I do it like this or should I put it up or down?" After raising four daughters, an "I don't know, ask your mom" doesn't fly.

"Wear it down," he answered. I again tugged at the binder and braced my head as it anything but slid off my hair. Bobby pins, I needed bobby pins. I checked every drawer, then every drawer in my bedroom and every one in my sister's unoccupied room. Not one. I was shocked. I rummaged and rummaged in every kind of thing that can be rummaged in, and just as I began to lose hope, it appeared: a single bobby pin. My practiced hand slipped it expertly into place, pinning my greasy bangs back from my face, and miraculously leaving my unwashed hair quite presentable indeed.

Stairs get easier every day, and I took them without holding the railing up to the kitchen. It smelled like spices and salt and I could feel the heat from the oven twenty feet away. I convinced my parents to let me open a door to cool down the room.

The doorbell rang for the first time just as my mom was setting out the last of the dirty shrimp and freshly baked pita crackers. I paused as greetings flew, waiting as our neighbor removed her boots, jacket, hat, scarf and mittens before rushing her for a hug. She was ushered in with the usual, what can I get you to drink?, and we made our way to the couches in front of the fire. "So what happened? Tell me everything," and I launched into my story for the first of many times that night.

The doorbell rang and knocks were heard several more times, each one more of an introduction than a request to enter. I tell my story to groups of two or three at a time as we mill about, shortening or lengthening it depending on how interested my audience seems and how much of their drinks they have left: anyone with an empty glass just keeps eyeing the uncorked wine bottles on the other side of the room.

My spiel consists of: I was diagnosed at age seven; I have simple partial seizures, my right hand clenches up and shakes but I'm still conscious; I underwent some monitoring back in November; there were two surgeries; first one to put in electrodes; monitored and reverse stimulated the electrodes to see what happened; took out grids and chunk of brain; I'm doing well; the end. I repeat it over and over, throwing in different anecdotes and jokes to change it up for me and for anyone listening who'd heard it before. I repeated over and over, but it was so good to see them that I didn't mind. Not at all.

Everyone brought appetizers and wine, and while I relegated myself to a can of San Pellegrino, the cheeses and fruits were wonderful. My side mullet was in full form and I was told that a girl at the grocery store in town has the same haircut but on purpose, at which I was more amused than surprised. I might have to visit that grocery store...

It had been a good day. I'd been feeling well with minimal headaches since that morning, though I did decide to take a preemptive oxycodone so the crowd and noise wouldn't set me off running for a dark room with a pillow to cover my ears. The swirling energy of friends celebrating permeated my being, lifting me up and fueling me. We talked and laughed and exchanged stories of the things that have happened since we saw each other last. At 6:30 I turned into a pumpkin, as promised, and everyone left, fixing the Saran Wrap on the dishes they'd brought, buttoning their coats

158

and courteously keeping their goodbye's to five minutes rather than the customary fifteen.

The smile plastered on my face continued on through the dinner and a movie my parents and I watched in bed, the blu ray player in my computer hooked up to their tv, an extra sheet spread across the comforter to catch any food that might fall off one of the five or so trays balanced precariously on the bed. To be clear, that's not a normal occurrence, there just wasn't an HDMI plug in the regular tv, so we had to use the one in their room... yes, we're turning into a mid-90's wholesome after-school sit com family. I'm not sure whether I'm supposed to shudder or laugh, but I'll choose the latter.

Like I've said before, every day is different, but I look back now and am amazed at all of the progress I've made over just the past three weeks. I can walk, I can eat, I can read and I can entertain. Now that I'm open for business as a dancing monkey, I'll have to put together a schedule for my show and tell gigs!

## Twitchy Legs II

After many nights of exceedingly restless sleep, I've found some solutions: stretch before bed, massage my calves and sleep on my left.

I called my neurosurgeon's nurse at Mayo and spoke with her about my legs. I didn't think it was a seizure problem, but I wanted to be absolutely positive. I told her that it usually starts about an hour after I fall asleep and wakes me up. The twitches are just that: twitches, not shaking, so don't last long at all. It happens in both legs, which is the main reason we believe it's not seizure related. It all started after I'd begun to go on longer walks and use my legs more. She thinks it's because of that, which makes sense to me. It's just my body getting used to moving around again after being sedentary so long. She said she would still talk to both the surgeon and my neurologist and would call me back if they were concerned, but that if I don't hear from her, it means there's nothing to worry about. So far I haven't heard and it's been a few days, so I'm not worried.

One of the things that I've found helps is relaxing my legs before going to sleep. I unroll my yoga mat and spend five to ten minutes stretching. I can't believe how tight they are after only a month of not stretching them regularly through Pilates or any post-workout cool down! I stretch every leg muscle that I know how to stretch and chop my calf muscles and thighs, which is quite unpleasant, though I attribute that to the energy there that needs to be released.

The other thing I've found to work is sleeping on my left. Maybe lying on my right hip has started to pinch some nerve; I'm not sure, but getting off of it helps calm down my legs. The problem with that is that I wake up the next morning with a splitting headache. I can fall asleep on my left and can stay there for a while, but the left side of my head is still too tender to sleep on for a whole night. Fortunately I still have quite a bit of oxycodone left, but it would be nice if I didn't have to use it anymore. Oh well, that will come. In the mean time, for the most part my legs are back to normal.

In addition to my legs getting better, I've been feeling great these days. I have my moments - this morning with the oxycodone - but each day I'm able to walk farther and function better. Most days, instead of a nap I just have some quiet time in bed reading or watching tv or a movie on my computer. It's nice not to need a nap every two hours; I feel like I can start to be part of society again. It's quite nice!


## Singing In My Head

I don't remember what season it was, but the air was temperate enough that I could get by with a light sweater.

I held my mom's hand as we crossed the mildly busy street and stepped onto the curb. I was three or four years old - again, I don't quite remember, but I wasn't in kindergarten yet. Still, though, to this day the memory is vivid.
We were running errands, my mom needed a few things. I think we'd just left the shoe repair store with the green and yellow sign that I've walked by a hundred times but probably been to twice since that day.

I was happy. It was a great day: I was out with my mom and I had a song stuck in my head. The song was going round and round, like a goldfish in its bowl. I was smiling, I do remember that, the contented smile of a child without a care in the world. The bounce in my step was the prelude to a skip. The melody was one that I'd made up and didn't have any words to go with it, but that was fine by me.

160

We passed a man on the sidewalk - probably just a college student from the school nearby, but at that age anyone over four feet tall was a grownup. He looked at me, puzzled but amused, and I smiled back as we kept walking. Just behind him was a woman - or maybe she was first... I'm not sure, but it doesn't matter. She wore the that's-so-cute-my-heart-is-melting look that I wore yesterday as I saw a toddler struggling to multi-task with a door and a straw. I loved being adored, but suspicion crept over me, not the dark cloud of suspicion that floats over grownups, but a light shadow. And it hit me. "Mom, was I singing out loud just now?" I asked, on the border between embarrassed and horrified.

"Yes," she said distractedly. I slowed in my tracks, and she turned back to me, "But that's okay, honey, I love it. It's very pretty," she soothed, smiling.

Ugh. I'd done it again. I always did that! I always started singing out loud when I'd meant it to just be in my head. Why didn't I notice? I sighed. My worry was that people would think it's annoying, and I didn't want to annoy anyone. I was distraught. The sudden mood swings of a child, able to feel just one emotion at a time - an unappreciated luxury, like nap time. But wait, logic prevailed. Mom likes it when I sing, she's the only one here, and I like to sing, so I'll sing!

I changed to a real song, one with words, probably off of my Raffi record. I sang out loud on purpose as my bounce turned into a skip.


**Spring and Recovery**

Recovery is kind of like spring: every day is wildly different, but even if it snows, you're still steadily on your way to summer. The metaphor falls apart there, since today I felt great and it snowed ten inches with two to eight more to go, but you get my point. Spring has always been my least-favorite season since it's such a tease. As a kid and as a borderline-grownup, I get so excited the first March day that the temperature spikes to thirty, leaving my coat at home and venturing outside in a sweatshirt. I fantasize about summer and how this year I'm actually gonna do all the things I had meant to do last year but never did - picnic in the park every weekend, buy a bike and remember how to ride without looking like a wobbly five year old, etc. I get so excited picturing myself in my folding lawn chair with the backpack straps and the pocket full of snacks, a book and a water bottle filled with wine, that when two days later it's hailing, I'm so disappointed that I miss the bigger picture. Recovery has been a lot like that. I conquer staircases one day and ride the high for another, but the day after that I wake up to a throbbing headache and have to be escorted down to the kitchen from my bedroom and, shortly after, back up to my room. It's easy to get discouraged when I'm really beginning to appreciate the true meaning of, "two steps forward, one step back." "Look at the big picture," is the only cliché I can think of right now that promotes keeping my chin up, but it's true. Panning the camera back isn't always easy, and sometimes you want to just wallow, which is totally valid, but only for about half an hour, at which point you need to pick yourself up. Sitting in your room feeling sorry for yourself does not do anything to propel you toward recovery.

Yes, it's easy for me to say this since I'm having such a great day that I've only taken three Tylenol and it's ten pm, but even without today, even if, like Friday, I'd taken eight Tylenol and two oxycodones, I haven't had a Percocet in weeks, and that's huge. I remember in the hospital ranking my pain higher than I like to remember and asking the nurses every half hour when I could take my next pain meds. I can't believe that was already a month ago. I've come so far since then. I've passed basic motor skills and intermediate speech abilities and I think the next leg of my journey will come to be endurance. I'll take longer walks, write more, go to more crowded areas, try to take two excursions in a day. See what happens. I'm tempted to close with some play on weather getting warmer and spring turning to summer, but everything that comes to mind sounds far too cheesy. Instead, I'll just say that thinking of recovery as spring, as a transition that's not smooth, that often feels like a rollercoaster that makes you nauseous, helps. It helps a lot.

## A Seed of Doubt

Every day I cross something off of the list of things I can't do. I can walk, I can climb stairs, I can go without prescription pain meds. I'm proud of each small accomplishment, every shuffle, step or leap forward, but within each one is a seed of doubt, a hesitation.

I remember the first time the ICU nurses made me sit up in my hospital bed: it was the morning after the second surgery. I woke up, still in so much pain but thankfully not nearly as much as the night before - maybe an eight. My parents were there, I think I remember seeing my dad by my

162

bed. They wore the scent of the recently terrified and each had a cup of coffee to stave off the exhaustion left behind after the initial euphoria of success had worn off. It took me a little longer to process: I didn't get the euphoria until the drive home from the hospital and it was another three days before the high wore off, leaving me more emotionally exhausted than I've ever been before.

Between the lingering anesthesia, the pain and all of the medication, my memory of that day is foggy and comes in snippets closer to the length of a video you'd take on your phone than a full-length feature film. Even then, I wouldn't swear many details on the Bible.

I wasn't sure if I was going to tell my parents about the night before, about lying on the table in recovery, writhing in pain and sobbing for what felt like, and turned out to be, hours. I knew I should, but I didn't want them to feel even worse for me than they did; they had enough worries, their daughter was in the hospital. They had been with me so completely by then, though, that there was no way I could hold out on them now. No, I would come clean. Later.

I doubt I ate any breakfast, or at least any to speak of. I was too weak. Maybe just a little something to help wash down the pills. My nurse came in after I had thrown in the meal towel and informed me that I had to sit up. Excuse me? "Thanks but no thanks," was the dad-ism from my childhood that rang in my ears. I was too weak to sit up and too tired to try. This was the first morning waking up without the snake coiling from my brain to a machine and I could tell my head felt lighter. I said I couldn't sit up and wanted to take a nap, but that didn't fly. My parents offered gentle words of encouragement to counteract the harsh orders from the nurse as she wrenched me upright. It felt awful. Nonetheless, I remained there as she and my dad, who'd taken my other arm and back to guide me up, lightened their grips until I was flying solo. It felt good to know that I was able to sit up and dangle my legs over the bed, but thirty seconds later I negotiated myself a nap.

When I woke up, somewhere between fifteen minutes and two hours later, I was told that it was time for the move from the ICU to the non-intensive neuro recovery floor below us. That meant I had to get into a wheelchair. I've blocked out most of the memory of moving from the bed to the chair and I'm not sorry about it. It was painful and exhausting and just generally unpleasant; like a spin class with bad music.

Someone wheeled me down the hallway toward the elevators as my parents trailed behind, carrying all of the pictures and good luck knick nacks I'd brought, the care packages and letters I'd received, the Fruity Pebbles we'd smuggled in and the colorful hand-made sign stating, "We Love Our Erica," that my sister had sent me. At the elevator bank, my dad snatched his iPhone out of his pocket and snapped a picture of me on my transition to the next phase of recovery, though in actuality I was pointing at the open elevator and giving him an irritated look for taking too long and almost making us miss it. That flattering picture ended up posted on the blog, of course.

I arrived in my new room shortly, after bumping over every tiny seam in the linoleum like the Princess and the Pea and desperately wanting my next pain killers. I made it to bed by the grace of God and fell asleep as soon as people stopped asking me to touch my finger to my nose, wiggle my numb toes and swallow-that-while-we-inject-this. That day was exhausting. Every tiny thing, every task, every interaction, hit me like a pillow in the face and required a one to three hour nap to recharge.

That was just under a month ago. Sometimes it feels longer ago than that, or rather I feel more removed from it, but most of the time it feels like it just happened. When I first came home I was still in rough shape, but I knew where I was going. Now, today, I have no idea. I was told three months, but it's only been one and I don't know how much more there is left to do. I know that's crazy, hell, I still can't sleep on my left cause it's too sensitive, but I can't quite figure out what my next goals need to be. I still feel out of it sometimes and I tire fairly easily, but for the most part I'm doing really well. That should be a good thing, and it is, but the hesitation shows itself and asks me, "what now?" I don't know. When am I considered healed? What happens then? Do I get a job and go back to work? These questions have been put on hold for the most part since I decided to have surgery, but the closer I get to "better" the more pause I give myself. Am I ready to be "better?" I'm inclined to answer no, but even though it's true, I know that part of me just wants to stay in my little limbo cocoon until I know what to do with my life. Is that something I should be reflecting on and thinking about, or is this a time when it's okay to disregard stresses and worries for a while?

Don't get me wrong, I'm so grateful that I've gotten to this point, it's just that it feels like a turning point, a blind corner, and I don't know what's coming up, let alone how to handle it. Am I gonna be able to handle "real life" and when is it supposed to start? What is the rest of my recovery going to be like? What does it entail? At this point I really have no idea and I don't suppose I will until I get there. I just remind myself: recovery is good but there's no reason to rush.

## A New Swimsuit and Three New T-Shirts!

The spoils of war! And by war, I mean exercise. And by exercise, I mean shopping. Today I went on by far my biggest excursion yet: the Mall of America. It was wonderful. Basing my estimation on the map of the stores visited, in which order they were visited, and the fact that the distance around one level of the rectangular-shaped mall is .57 miles, I can confidently say that I walked at least a mile and a half today. A mile and a half!! Getting out and being around people was great. I don't mind my healing cocoon, but it's nice to get out. I'd been a little nervous about the noise and crowd and too many stimuli, but the extra oxycodone and nausea pills I packed in my purse ended up staying there. I kept thinking back to the times at the hospital when I had to take a nap to recover from talking more than five minutes with someone who had a stringent voice. We've come a long way, baby.

There is much more I could say, mostly re-wording my astonishment at the pace of my healing that I've talked about before, but I walked a mile and a half today, so I'm going back to sleep.

But first, one correction: the title of this entry should be, A New Swimsuit, Three New T-Shirts and a Build-a-Bear! I got to make a Build-a-Bear today at the Mall with a dear friend of mine whom I've known since first grade. We swapped furry friends as we registered them and made them birth certificates - he named my bear Hope. I thought it was very fitting. Hope.

## Mission: Patience

I stood up from the table in the kitchen looking over the snowy back yard that has officially been dubbed "Erica's office." Soothing music from an artist whose name I couldn't guess floated behind me as I walked barefoot into the living room, carrying a stack of letters waiting to be addressed and stamped. I spotted the address book next to a roll of stamps on my dad's desk and padded down the two carpeted steps toward it. I've been writing thank you cards for the past two days and my neck and back were sore from hunching over each folded card with a pen that kept running out of ink. I walked with my back straight and head in line with my spine to pacify the grumbling muscles. I looked up at the ceiling, stretching my neck, and my knees almost gave out. My legs turned to rubber and my arms threatened to follow. The blood in my head rushed in some direction, I couldn't say if it was in or out, but all I could think was that I was too weak to stay standing; I was about to collapse. The edges of my vision turned blurry, but right in the middle of the forming tunnel was the large, black desk chair. I bee-lined toward it, losing altitude but determined to make it. I angled my body slightly sideways and slid onto the plush, rolling savior. I made it. I exhaled. I haven't fallen once since the surgery and though a carpet would be the ideal place on which to try, I had no intention of starting now. I'm not taking nearly as many pain killers as I used to, but my head is still just this side of eggshell.

In the past month - I can't believe it's already been a month - I've progressed by leaps and bounds, but I still get terrible head rush almost every time I stand up. Usually I can grab on to a counter or table or dresser or arm, but sometimes I need to just sit down as quickly as I can, especially when I'm on the stairs. It becomes irritating; not quite frustrating, but irritating. I know it's something that will take time, that will go away on its own when it's ready, but I still keep trying to figure out what causes it so I can skip a few steps and get rid of it. I'm still working on resigning myself to the "marathon, not a sprint" truth. I'll get there.

In the meantime, I've found that I have more stamina every day - most days I don't even take naps anymore! I walked all around the Mall of America without passing out and having to be fireman-carried back to the car. Granted, I was shot for the rest of that day and a fair amount of the next, but it was worth it. Yesterday, despite the hangover in my legs, I was able to get out and ride 45 minutes to my therapist for a full one hour session! When I got back, I took a little quiet time and some lunch before one of the pastors from my church came over to visit. In summary, I had an excursion, talked about my feelings for an hour, and then talked about church for an hour, all without a nap or caffeine! I spent the rest of the day in bed, but still.

Then we come to today. My mission, should I choose to accept it, is to attend a thousand-person banquet tonight in downtown Minneapolis.

That's a lot of people. Pros: I'll get to cheer on my mom as she receives a lawyer award, I'll get to snap a picture of her horrified face if they put part of her pre-taped interview on the jumbotron and I'll get to dress up. Cons: that's a lot of people, each having a conversation as they scrape their many forks and knives across their plates. I'm not sure if I can handle that much stimulation. The whole thing will realistically last about two and a half hours, and if I need to leave early, I can just slip away and grab a cab back to St. Paul. I'm signed up to go, but the plan is for me to decide close to the last minute based on how I feel this afternoon. As the clock reads ten to one, it is officially afternoon. Right now, I'm torn. I don't know. I really want to be there to support and cheer on my mom, but just thinking about it makes me exhausted. Maybe what I'll do is take a shower and get dressed for it, and if I'm feeling okay, I'll go, otherwise, if I'm spent from just getting ready, I'll stay home. Yeah. That sounds like a good plan.

It's hard to be kind-of-recovered. At times, I feel like I can do almost anything, but then I try to actually do it and I just can't. It's not as much of a tease as it is a deception; my body is conning me. But again, "it's a marathon, not a sprint." I should write that out on my mirror, either with a label maker set to a fun font, or in lipstick. Either way, I need to keep reminding myself that there are some things I'm just not ready for and that that's okay. Patience has never been one of my virtues, but neither has the ability to be dependent, and I've learned that over the past months. I can learn patience. That will be my next mission.


## Middle School

My hair was dry enough to work with after being twisted up in a scarf and secured with a hat on top since the customary towel turban was too heavy. My ear piece was still in my ear as I applied my mascara, but I was going to take it out and switch off the Bluetooth toggle on my phone to save the battery. I began to screw the mascara wand back into its holster when Ke$ha interrupted The Big Bang Theory playing on my computer, informing me that the party doesn't start until she arrives. Also that my phone was ringing. It was my sister, calling to hear and tell stories and swap nuggets of wisdom. She knew most of what was going on with me from the blog, but I was able to come up with more, talking about my feelings and life in general, hearing about her classes and her daughters' snow days. We talked about the struggles life presents, the times when you feel like they'll never end, and the times when you suddenly realize that you came out on top. We talked about my plan for the next year or two, what I want to do, what I want to accomplish, etc. And then it struck me: being in your twenties is a lot like being in middle school. You don't really know where you fit in in the world and there's an awkwardness and acute self-awareness that follows you around; classes are harder, you have more homework and have to learn to juggle and multi-task; you have a new favorite subject every day, deciding that you want to be a doctor, no, a painter, no, a mathematician; you're expected to grow up.

I've had my fair share of struggles in the past five years, but who hasn't? What matters is what you do with those struggles. I used mine to learn about myself and extrapolate that to understand other people. I got the strength to work through depression and anxiety problems when I realized that my default status had always been happy, and that that's a gift worth fighting to get back. Anorexia I developed in part as a control mechanism, a way of bringing just a little order to the chaos and uncertainty in my life. Later on, it was times of instability that caused it to come back. When I figured that out, I gained a powerful weapon: foresight. I learned how to check in with and monitor myself. I also learned that I can't always rely on my own mind to make the right decisions and that it's important for me to let people in and ask them for help. Oddly enough, the struggle I lived with the longest was the one whose lessons took the longest to sink in. From an early age, my epilepsy showed me the world in a different light: I understood what it was like to be different, to have a health limitation that my friends didn't. I was more aware and more sensitive to other people who were different, and often when I heard their stories, I realized how lucky I was. I could ride a bike, water ski, go to summer camp, go build houses in Guatemala, hike the Inca trail, be on the swim team, go to college. I thanked God every day for how blessed I was. The only lesson I didn't learn was that I didn't have to do it alone; it's okay to ask for help. "Asking for help doesn't mean you failed, it just means your not in it alone," is a quote I heard recently that stuck with me. Okay, Josh Duhamel says it in Life as We Know It, but still, it's profound, and, more importantly, it's true. I didn't get that before. It took a team of doctors literally opening up my brain for me to understand the truth of that and I'm so glad I finally get it. I asked for help with a burden I'd largely carried alone for eighteen years, and it ended up being one of the hardest and best decisions of my life.

## Not Quite Polka-Dots

Little white specks unevenly cover the left shoulder of my navy blue sweatshirt. They center just above my shoulder proper, spreading out from an increasingly solid-colored Ground Zero like a sunburst over my collarbone and back. The left side of my head, these days coated with almost three-quarters of an inch of hair, itches to high Heaven and back, and every time I scratch it, more white specs fall silently, like snow in the night.

Winter here is drier than hangover mouth, and without sufficient hair to coat my scalp with hair oil, it becomes dry and flaky. The right side of my head is fine for the most part, but it's home to a foot and change of thick, curly hair. I've tried massaging my scalp in the shower and saturating the peach fuzz on the left side with super-hydrating conditioner, but without its former protection, it's no use; my left scalp is too vulnerable to the elements.

Last night, I sat in bed reading a book on the virtues of meditation and could not for the life of me stop itching my head every minute or two. Exasperated, I surveyed my room for anything that might make it stop, and suddenly, like a beacon of light, my eyes landed on a tall, white bottle of Lubraderm. Why hadn't I thought of that before? It's not as though I'm going out for a beauty pageant - hell, even a cheesy night club - one of these days, so a little greasy peach fuzz is really not a problem. What a fabulous idea! I palmed the flat above the nozzle and pumped three times, filling the hand below it with a generous amount of blessed, creamy white soothing power. Full of lotion, I brought my left hand to my head and wiped a gob onto my hair. I massaged it into my thirsty scalp until all that remained was a thin film between my fingers. Ahhhhh. I sighed contentedly and wondered again why this hadn't occurred to me sooner. Ah well, I knew the magic secret now, which was all that mattered. I kept the plastic bottle with blue trim next to my bed in case I woke up scratching my head again and finally, finally got some rest.

## Excursion Hangover

I haven't had a drink since the surgery, but I'm discovering a new type of hangover that has become more and more prevalent as I've become more and more active: the excursion hangover. Last night I got nine hours of sleep, and even though all I've done today is eat and watch a USA Network show on OnDemand, I'm exhausted. So incredibly exhausted, and with a headache to match. The cause is not from champagne, wine or drinks with little umbrellas, it's from singing, and it's completely worth it. My eyelids are drooping heavily, my mind is working at half speed and there's a shooting pain through my head, but Mozart's Requiem floats through me, its melodic beauty filling my body and dampening my ails.

My parents yelled up from the kitchen to hurry up. "One sec! I'm coming!" I replied, picking up my bottle of Fast Relief Tylenol gel caps. I popped off the child-proof top and shook two into my palm. Half a glass of water sat on my nightstand and I grabbed it as I tossed the painkillers down the hatch. I glanced quickly around the room to make sure I wasn't forgetting anything. Music, check, Kindle, check, cell, check, nausea pills just in case, check. I carefully went down the stairs as quickly as my cautious feet would take me. One jacket, scarf, hat and pair of gold flats later, I shuffled over the icy driveway and deposited myself in the back seat.

As we backed out of the driveway, I sat up straight and leaned slightly to the left until I could see myself in the rear view mirror and steadily applied dark red lipstick: Lancôme's Sugared Maple to be exact. This was a big moment and I wanted to look my best. Every year, my high school holds a concert that includes a large mass piece. In addition to all of the student choirs and the orchestra, alumni, parents, teachers and community members are invited to join the Community Chorale. This year, the piece they're performing is Mozart's Requiem - hands down my favorite piece I've ever sung. It's beautiful and it's challenging, both emotionally and physically. I won't be around for the actual performance since it's not until late April, but the director, whom I've sung for since eighth grade and whom I consider a friend, said that I would be welcome to join the rehearsals while I'm still in town. The excitement running through my veins made me jittery, like I'd had three cups of stale coffee before giving in and draining a grande non-fat latte. I held the music book in my hand, the songs already circling my head, I can't believe I'm doing this! Singing a piece like that for a two and a half hour rehearsal with fifty other singers belting at the tops of their voices was to be my greatest undertaking yet.

When we pulled up in front of the school, I reminded my mom that I might have to call her to pick me up early if it got to be too much. She reassured me that she would keep her phone on her, using the same voice spoken to nervous kindergartners on their first day of school. I shuffled cautiously to the entrance, took a deep breath and went in.

Most of the chairs were empty as I walked the perimeter toward what I assumed would fill out to be the soprano section and chose a seat in the front. I unzipped my big puffy coat and draped it over the plastic chair along with my scarf. I dropped my purse by my feet after double checking that my phone was on silent. I left my hat on.

Upon arrival, my director greeted me with a warm hug, asking how I was, good, healing well, how are you? I told her I might have to go early if it gets to be too much and that I would likely stay sitting most of the times we were supposed to stand up. She understood completely and said that was no problem at all.

Five or ten minutes after me, the bulk of the singers arrived, taking off hats and gloves as they walked in, chatting as they stood around the card table in the corner, waiting to get coffee or tea or a name tag. I watched them until I felt self-conscious, the only one not talking to anybody, and turned back around to study my music. A girl who graduated two years ahead of me came over and took the chair next to me and we gave the customary, "Wow! It's been so long! It's great to see you!" and filled each other in on our lives. I had someone to talk to – I must not be a social pariah!

Greeted, caffeinated and seated, it was finally time to start rehearsal. This was it, it was go time. Moment of truth. And then the most magical thing happened: I opened my mouth. I took a deep breath, held my music up so I could see the director, and something inside me broke free. My soul rushed out of me, so eager to show the world that it was free, that it was singing. Its song joined fifty other voices, echoing off each other in a joyous release. Though not easy, or particularly sturdy, I stood with the rest of the class; I was too happy to hear my body's protests, but that was fine.

We ran through a whole movement before stopping to go back and tackle trouble spots. I relished the last note, sustaining it as long as I could, but I kept running out of breath. Though everyone else stayed standing, I sat down as we rustled through our music books to and from rehearsal letters A through Z, running and rerunning this part or that. I noticed as I sang that I hardly had half the breath capacity that I used to. I'm sure it will return as I get stronger, but for the time being I feel like I'm hyperventilating after each measure.

We ran the movement again from the beginning and I started to stand up but thought better of it. As we sang, the director pointed at her cheek bones and yelled, "sing here!" I manipulated the sound within me and aimed it at my cheek bones, where I knew it would land in my sinus cavities. It did. The sound reverberated in my sinuses, throwing a clear song out of me but leaving my head vibrating. I felt a little like a cartoon character whose head was clunked by two symbols and kept vibrating, even their irises going back and forth in their whites like they're watching a tennis volley. I had to pause, catch my breath, hold my head with both hands until it stopped moving. I stuck it out through sheer will power for just two more bars until we reached the end.

The rehearsal lasted two and a half hours, and though my shaky insides protested at mile marker two hours, I kept singing. I couldn't bring myself to leave yet, it felt too good to stop.

On the way out, my director stopped me and asked how it went: "It was amazing! I didn't stand up for the whole time, but I sang all of it! Now I'm gonna go home and sleep for three days." And I did.

March, 2011

## A Tickle in My Throat

The past couple mornings I've woken up with a sore throat. My mom swears by EmergenC, so I dissolve one in a glass of grapefruit juice, watching the lemon-flavored powder fizz as I try to stir out the clumps. It doesn't take to the juice as well as Benefiber, and I have to use my spoon to squish the clumps against the side of the glass to break them up into grainy, vitamin C sand. I take a deep breath and down the juice in three gulps; I don't want it to congeal before I get a chance to drink it. Setting the glass, empty but for the spoon used to stir it, on the table, I hope that I'm not coming down with something.

I remember the months going up to the surgery, and being so scared that I would get sick and they wouldn't operate on me. I was terrified of anything that would preclude the doctors from going ahead with my surgery. I tried not to dwell on it, to take care of myself without the gnawing fear, but of course it was still there. How could it not be? Waiting on a surgery like that, waiting to see if maybe, just maybe, your life could be forever changed, there's no way you can stay calm and put together all the time.

Five weeks removed, I'm not scared anymore; a cold would be more of an inconvenience. What does make me nervous is that, historically, my seizure threshold is lower when I'm sick. The possibility that no one would operate on me as a catalyst for fear has been replaced by the possibility that it didn't work. It's been over a month and I haven't had a single seizure. I've done my best to stay away from anything that could act as a trigger, but any time that my right hand feels weak, my heart starts beating faster and my breath gets shallow and quick. On the surface, I know that I'm still getting function back in the hand that once couldn't hold a fork, but underneath, my stomach churns.

An hour later, the pain in my throat is back. I heat up water for some tea, but I doubt it'll work. Maybe I should take a nap. I had a big day yesterday: two excursions, one Skype appointment and a family friend over for dinner. Each activity was fun and I enjoyed myself very much, but it was the first time in weeks that I took two naps in one day.

Yesterday I didn't write, mostly because if I wasn't busy, I was sleeping. I glanced at my computer, seeing it sideways from my pillow, but couldn't summon the energy. I always feel guilty when I don't blog. It's really not necessary for me to feel guilty, I have no legitimate reason to, but I do anyway. I was just so tired. I'm tired again today, a hangover from my big day yesterday, but writing feels nice. It always does, unless I'm falling asleep on my keyboard, which has happened more than once...

Anyway, that's what's in my head today. Fairly inconsequential thoughts swirling around, leaving patterns in their wakes while I drift off to sleep.


## Back Up to Five

I woke up this morning at a five on the pain scale, maybe even six for a little bit. A searing pain... is that a thing? "Searing pain?" Or am I just stringing together words from different sayings? I don't remember. Either way, "searing" is the word that comes to mind as I try to describe the shooting line of pain that woke me up an hour before my alarm. I tried to go back to sleep, but I couldn't. I just laid there. That's another word: laid vs. lay vs. lie, I never really know when to use which, so I just guess. I should look that up one of these days. Anyway, shortly after that, my mom came in to my room to check on me before she left for work. She asked how I was feeling, but I just looked up at her, my eyes mostly closed to the light pouring in from the hallway, dreading the vibrations that would fill my head as I spoke. I replied with some form of, "my head really hurts." She walked over to my bedside, a mask of loving concern on her face as she reached down and held my wrist. I told her that I'd just taken two Tylenols and that hopefully they would kick in soon. She put her hand on my forehead and I maneuvered it, testing its temperature, until her warm palm lifted away and her cold fingers rested just above my eyes. It hurt so bad. She asked me if I wanted a cold pack and took my lack of answer as a yes. She left and walked downstairs to the kitchen, stopping on the way to tell my dad that I wouldn't be driving him to the airport this afternoon. I felt disappointed because I'd been looking forward to driving again, but I knew she was probably right; even if I were feeling better, I should start by driving on empty roads, not the highway.

Mom came back up the creaking stairs, carrying a freezer-sized Ziploc full of ice cubes and wrapped in a brown dishtowel with a fall leaf pattern on it. She placed it on the left side of my head as I lay on my right. I took it and moved it into place, trying unsuccessfully to balance it so I wouldn't have to hold the cold pack as it covered itself in condensation. Oh well, holding it was better than not having it. Mom went to work, promising to call and check in. I held my ice pack in place and drifted into a three-quarter sleep. The cold felt good. Great, even.

When it started to melt and I could feel the drops of cold water slide from my hairline down my neck, catching in my t-shirt, an oversized, white welcome greeter, I lifted off the cold pack and gently dropped it onto the floor. The neck of my shirt was wet and I cringed inwardly every time it touched my skin as I rearranged myself in the bed. I looked at the green, digital numbers on the 1970s, brown alarm clock that sat on the other side of the room and decided to give myself fifteen more minutes for the headache to die down before I would give up and take an oxycodone. But fifteen minutes later, I pushed back my covers and stood up in stages, finding that a five turned into a six the farther I got from horizontal. I could feel my face arrange itself into a look of pain and brought a hand to my head. The dresser stands only four feet away, making the pharmacy on top of it easy to reach. I hadn't taken an oxycodone in well over a week and it pained me to push down and turn the child-proof bottle top. I slid one small, white pill into my hand and eyed the half glass of water on my nightstand, pausing before reaching out to it. I had pills to take, and since I was up, I should just take them all. I opened each bottle in turn, shaking one of this kind and two of that into my hand. I threw the total seven into my mouth and gulped them down with the room temperature water. I stood for just a moment to make sure they all went down before climbing back into bed. I picked up my Droid with its purple half-cover (I broke the front half at a bagel shop a few months ago) and re-set the alarm for 10:30 - a half-hour away. I figured it would take about thirty minutes for the oxycodone to kick in.

Half-way through my sleep, my mom called. How's your headache? Same. Are you still in bed? Yes. Is your dad there? Just left, but he'll be back in a couple hours. I'm sorry, honey. Thanks; me too. Did you end up taking an oxycodone? Yeah, I just did. Okay, good.

It hurt to talk, so I didn't linger or chat. I explained that I planned to wake up in fifteen minutes, when, hopefully, the resignedly-taken narcotics had started to work. She paused; "I wonder if we should take you to the hospital..." Why? "You haven't had a headache like this in a while. What if your brain is bleeding? Are you having any neurological symptoms on your right side?" No, I'm okay.

We performed a neuro exam anyway. I wiggled my fingers and toes, wagged my tongue from side to side, held out my hands with my palms

176

both up and down. She felt better when I told her I was able to open all of my pill bottles with no trouble.

With an, "I love you," we hung up and I went back to sleep.

I awoke again with my phone alarm singing me a Jack Johnson song that started quietly and got progressively louder - one of the alarm settings I'd turned on. I slid my finger across the face of the phone to dismiss it and touched the email icon. My eyelids were heavy as I scrolled through the emails, separating the bad junk from the junk with coupons I might use from the legitimate emails. I picked up my computer and opened my Blogger dashboard just as my dad called me. We went through the same conversation pattern as mom, but instead of brain bleeding and a phone-conducted exam, he substituted that he would be home in a few hours and planned to take a cab to the airport. "I'm sorry I can't drive you," I added.

"Don't worry, honey. I'm fine. I just want you to get better." Again, an, "I love you" ended the vibrations that radiated from my sinus cavities.

My head was feeling a little better, so I spent an hour and a half blogging in bed before deciding it was time for breakfast.


**The Red Sea**

Lately, my scar has been reminding me of the Red Sea as it parted for Moses. A long, thin, red line runs from the back of my head, straight down the continental divide at the top before veering left an inch before the hairline and ending at my left temple. Flanking the scar are two long stretches of bald, one on each side. I don't know why, but I keep thinking of the Red Sea parting along my scar; rather, the site of my scar and the two bowling lanes that run down its sides. Strangely, Moses must have gained weight on the way, because at the top of my head the part is almost twice as wide. I'm not sure why...

I've been putting scar-reducing lotion on the fault line to help it heal and shrink, but so far I haven't noticed any difference when it comes to the hair that keeps falling out. I rub my index finger in the pot of solid lotion, the heat from my hand melting it like a candle. I have to look in the mirror to make sure I'm applying it in the right place, not in a patch of perfectly good, if buzzed, hair. I rub the lotion onto my scalp, trying to help, and even though I take my hand away and see that it's covered with little, dark brown hairs, each time I'm still sure it'll work. Soon enough; soon enough.

## Pink, Sparkles and Frills

I sat on the twin bed in the Aunt Alice room, tracing the blue and white floral patterns of the quilt with my finger. The Aunt Alice room was really just the guest room, but my Great Aunt Alice always stayed there when she came to visit, so we called it her room. She was really old, older than my grandma. She smelled like old people, but she always had lots of stories about when she was a little girl like me. Her refrigerator was made out of a wooden box! And when it was cold in the winter, she and grandma would put rocks in the fire to make them hot and then put them by their feet in their beds to keep them warm.

Aunt Alice wasn't visiting that day, but I was sitting in her room with my mom. I watched my finger as it outlined each flower, leaf and stem on the bedspread. I didn't want to look at mom cause I knew she'd ask me what was wrong and I didn't wanna tell her. I didn't wanna talk about it, I just wanted to forget about it. When I was done tracing everything I could reach, I folded my hands and looked at my lap.

We were going somewhere, and mom asked me what I wanted to wear. I'd been thinking a lot at school that day, watching the other kindergartners on the playground, half of the girls choosing the navy blue jumpers over navy blue uniform pants. The boys always spilled their lunch on their white polo shirts and got dirt and grass stains on them at recess, but mine were always clean. I didn't play in the mud with the boys. Yuck! Boys are so weird.

Still looking down, I dropped my head to the right, my ear fusing to my shrugged shoulder in an, "I'm embarrassed and don't want to do this with you right now" fashion. Normally, I loved picking out clothes, but my little, pigtailed head was full of doubts and insecurities.

"I wanna wear a dress," I answered quietly. I always wanted to wear a dress. The more frills, the better. Pink, too. It was my favorite color. I had a pair of pink jellies with sparkles in them, and they were sooooo pretty, but it was too cold out. I had a pair of sparkly ruby red slippers like Dorothy in The Wizard of Oz, and they were warmer cause the toes were closed

178

on them, unlike the jellies, so maybe I could wear those. I'd ask mom about that.

I had never told mom why I always had to wear dresses. I was embarrassed about it; I didn't want her to laugh or even try to be nice about it, cause that still wouldn't change anything. I had a really low voice. When I talked, I sounded like a boy. I hated it!! Every time I opened my mouth to say something, it sounded like a boy talking! I had to make sure no one thought I was a boy, make sure that everyone knew I was a girl, so I had to wear dresses. It was the only solution. The girlier, the better. Dresses, frills, bows, sparkles, pink, the whole shebang. Nikky F.'s mom would braid her hair that special way that made it look like the braid started at the top of her head - she called it a "french braid" - but my mom didn't know how to do that, so I had to have a regular braid that didn't start until it got off my head. Pigtails looked better than that, so most of the time I would opt for those instead. Or maybe just a high, side ponytail with a binder that had those little, colored balls on the end. I didn't know how to use them myself, even though I'd tried on my little sister more than once, but my mom could do it.

Mom asked if I wanted to wear the green dress with the little flowers on it and the ruffle at the bottom. I loved that dress, it was really pretty. I said yeah. No one would think I was a boy if I wore that.

Twenty years later, I stand in front of my mirror, turning left so I can just see the long, shiny hair that cascades past my collarbone. It's so pretty, so long. So feminine. I pause, a wistful look in my eyes, something just shy of a smile on my mouth. It's gonna take at least three years for me to get my hair this long again. I close my eyes and turn right, preparing myself for what I know I'm about to see. I gather my strength and look again to the mirror. The hair on the left side of my head isn't even an inch long yet. It grows in funny directions, leaving what looks like bald spots in the places where it changes from growing right to growing up, growing up to growing left. Front and center, featured so boldly I can easily imagine it surrounded my neon signs in the shape of arrows, is The Scar. It runs right down the middle of my head, veering left just before my forehead to curve behind my temple and complete its trace of the incision made only five weeks ago; the incision that changed the course of my life.

I'm proud of my battle wound, a sign of the fight I chose and won against the odds. I'm proud of the strength I found within myself and the strength I was given by others. I'm proud to be part of this human race that is able to love so fiercely and hold so gently people they hardly know. But still, my head flops to the side and my ear fuses to my shrugged shoulder as I emit an almost-silent whine, lamenting the return of a long-overcome fear: I'm gonna look like a boy.

In just a couple weeks, I'm going to cut my beautiful curls to match the mannish buzz cut on the masculine side of my Victor/Victoria head.

It's never gonna grow back and I'm gonna look like a man, is the thought that goes through my head like a marquee. My solution: same as it was last time, pink, sparkles and frills. Maybe not to the same degree as when I was five, but definitely with the same intention. I'll wear pink, lavender, light green; all those colors that girls - I mean, women - like. I'll buy clothes with hints of ruffles and flowers on them. I'll use the gift card I got for Christmas to get that swimsuit with the ruffles and eyelets. I'll wear a little more than my usual amount of makeup when I go out and I'll always wear earrings. And maybe a necklace, too. I don't want to look gaudy or trashy, but I want to make sure no one thinks I'm a boy. I don't have grass stains on my white shirt, and I certainly didn't play in the mud during my lunch break. I'm not going to start now.

## Without a Paddle

I just got off the phone with COBRA. Apparently, they lost my payments for January, February and March. As of January 1st, 2011, they terminated my health coverage. The woman said that it's not uncommon for them to accidentally post payments to the wrong account, but there's nothing she can do. Now, unless I can track down each check, I'm up shit creek without a paddle. I can hardly breathe.

## Typing With My Eyes Closed

The snow is melting. The table on the back porch, so recently covered in a tower of snow two feet high or taller, is now home to a wet patch of melting white the size of a serving dish. I watch it through the french doors that separate us, the barrier between fifty degrees and seventy, and can almost see drops of water dripping, dripping, through the slated tabletop. The chairs, once hidden completely, are exposed all the way down to the seat. The mounds on their laps grow smaller by the minute, gravity work-

180

ing with heat to force their osmosis through the wide mesh to the snow-padded stone floor.

Inside, my nose is cold, but I've turned off the switch-on fireplace behind me. I put a hand on my face to warm it, but the rest of me, for once in jeans instead of sweatpants, is just right. My eyes are drooping, tired from worrying about insurance and hurting from staring at a computer screen all day. Too much backlit reading. I should probably take a break soon. Maybe a nap. I haven't napped for the past two days. I've skipped my nap before, but always substituting some quiet time in bed, reading a book or watching tv on my computer. The past two days have been too busy. Today has been busy, too, but I feel the comfort of sleep coming over me; I feel myself being wrapped in a cocoon and pulled to bed. I'm hungry, I haven't had lunch yet and it's almost three, so I try to resist sleep, I try to resist the force that wants to lift me off my feet and carry me to bed. Which leftovers in the fridge would be the easiest to heat up and the quickest to eat? The turkey burger looks good, but it would really be better if I cut up a tomato and some cucumber to go with it. I'll do that later. Maybe that grain mom cooked that's supposed to be really good for you... I can't remember the name...

I type with my eyes closed, no longer able to force the lids to attention. My head lowers to the table, I'm typing upside down with my eyes closed... I'll spell check it before I post. I'm just so tired.

I haven't yet resolved the problem with COBRA, but I'm working on it, and with a friend who does HR law and a mom who's a litigator, I take comfort in the fact that I have good people on my side. It turns out that Aetna is the one who's in breach. In my Benefits Appeal to COBRA, I have to include that, but I also have to convince TriNet, the HR contractor, that I was incapacitated in January, which I was. Hell, I'm still incapacitated at times - like right now. Wow, dealing with this insurance is beyond stressful. I did some research and it turns out no other providers will take me because of my pre-existing conditions and the number and prices of name brand drugs I take. COBRA is really my only option until I get a new job that can give me health coverage. Good health insurance is my deal-breaker when it comes to finding a new job.

Mom and I worked last night on a draft of an appeal, which our friend edited and adjusted today. Tonight I'll fix up the final draft and send it. Pray for me. I need this to work. If it doesn't, we have to take it to court, and if

I lose... I can hardly think about it. I'll be without insurance. I need a nap. This stress is pulling all of my energy from me.

## Forgiving, Accepting and Moving Forward

How was I blessed with such amazing parents?

Tonight I put the green, Glassy Babies votive on the round, glass, living room table as I set it for dinner. I've been lighting three small, clear tea lights every night, but this afternoon I saw the green one and thought I'd substitute it for one of my usuals. It's colorful, and I was feeling in the mood for a touch of color.

We made it through the rounds of dish passing, take some broccoli, pass to the right, take some salad, pass to the right, take some shwarma, pass to the right, in easy conversation punctuated by lifting and dropping serving spoons and scraping knives and forks. I had finished half of my dinner when my dad asked, "So what's going on with this insurance thing?"

Color started to slowly creep into my face as my heart began to sink. My mom and I tag-teamed our way through a short-hand version of the past few days: paying five hundred dollars for one prescription at Walgreens, calling Aetna, calling TriNet, talking to mom, talking to Julie (an HR lawyer friend in Boulder), calling Aetna, calling TriNet, asking Eve in Denver to check the empty mail box in my apartment just to be sure, going through the paperwork from COBRA, talking to mom, talking to Julie, finding out the appeal process, drafting a benefits appeal request, sending it to the Benefits Appeal Committee, waiting, trying to be calm but often failing.

"How did this happen?" he asked, shocked that responsible Erica and anal retentive Becky could let slip a health insurance payment right as I was going into surgery. Believe me, I'm shocked too.

I stammered a minute, trapped like a mouse in my head, trying to find somewhere to throw the blame but unable, "I messed up." It's the truth. I messed up big, badly. I think about it, how stupid I was to bring this upon myself. My sinking heart hit the ocean bottom. Shame and embarrassment mixed with more bitter ingredients and spread itself like sour, brown paste over my insides, drowning all of the new self-confidence I'd went through

182

so much to find, worked so hard to build. I hate myself when I think about it. How dumb can I be? I completely deflated.

On Thursday, the cleaners came. I had just found out about my insurance being discontinued and was trying to figure out why. I'd been growing more and more panicked, and by the time I heard the side door opening, I was blinking back tears of frustration and fear. I pulled it together by the time they climbed the half staircase to the kitchen and said my "hola"s and "¿Cómo está?"s, I grabbed my things and all but ran upstairs and shut myself in my room.

I pulled the blue file folders out of my drawer and splayed out their contents on the hardwood floor. Each page entitled, "Description of Benefits", was itemized, showing every service, every pill, every piece of gauze, with a total at the end that I used to laugh at, so grateful that I wasn't the one who had to foot the bill. But this time... The calculator app on my phone worked double time summing every dollar, every penny, until I hit Enter. My heart was racing and I was in a cold sweat. I... but that's... but I'm... oh my God... what have I done??

Not only did I hate myself, I was sure that my parents would feel the same. How could they feel anything but disappointment in me? Their opinion of me would never be the same, they wouldn't trust me. A big, black stain was growing, tainting this event that has been surrounded by love and courage, dark ink seeping through the fabric of hope, happiness and closeness that has covered us since my first incision. What would happen to that? My parents and I had become so close, would all that work come undone? I was terrified of what they would think, terrified at what kind of low esteem I would be held.

I snapped back to dinner, to the conversation at hand, bracing myself for the unraveling that I had already begun to mourn, when my mom said, "Honey, it's okay." What? "Well, it's actually a big deal, but it's okay." Huh? "Everybody makes mistakes. This is a huge one, but it's not that bad: you weren't driving a barge not paying attention and hit a bridge, killing a bunch of people as their cars just drove off it like a cliff. You didn't hurt anybody, you didn't hurt yourself."

"So, my consolation is that I didn't kill anyone?" I asked.

My mom laughed, "Yes. Hey, one thing I've learned in life is not to waste time punishing yourself. Beating yourself up isn't productive, it's not going to change what already happened. Don't spend time thinking about whose fault it might have been, just accept that there's a problem and focus on fixing it."

She didn't hate me. Neither of them did. I had been so scared that they would and so sure that when they looked at me, all I would see in their eyes was disappointment. I'm not a parent, but I think I'm starting to figure out a few things: when you're a parent, the only thing you want for your kids is for them to be happy, and you would go to the ends of the earth and back to make that happen. At least that's what I've gathered. Tonight, at every lull, every silence, I felt awful about myself, but I could feel my mom's eyes on me, and she would ask me what was wrong. I looked at her with a face that said, "Are you kidding me?", but all she did was comfort me. I lost a few tears when I got up to clear the table and carried plates to the kitchen. She hugged me in the pink fleece jacket that she got ten years ago, and despite the two inches I have on her and the frailness I see more of lately, I felt better. I'm supposed to be kind of a grown-up now, but when my mom tells me everything is going to be alright, I believe it's true.

## Mourning a Loss

I miss coffee. I miss it so much. My terrible but wise decision to cut caffeine out of my life has left a gaping hole in my soul; an empty, dark void that used to be filled with black liquid. I smell stale coffee, cold after sitting it its pot for four hours, and I'm sucked back into a world filled with vibrant colors and not a drooping eyelid in sight. I feel a gravitational pull toward the kitchen cabinet that holds those blessed, white, ceramic vessels, I want to watch the dark liquid undulate in the cup as it's poured into itself, a waterfall of a wakeful day to come. I dig my heels into the floor, though low on traction, to hold myself back and with great effort tear my eyes away from the scene.

I put the room-temperature pot and its cold coffee down, placing it where it belongs: the coffee pot, not my hand. I turn back to my cup of herbal tea, sitting innocently on the counter, waiting for me to give up, resign myself to my uncaffeinated fate. The pink contents smell of hibiscus and are a poor substitute for the taste my lips remember from so many mornings with breakfast, afternoon pick-me-ups, evening study sessions. Coffee has punctuated my life since senior year of high school, defining my hang outs, being a place where I can catch up with friends or catch up with a book, providing a safe activity for first dates when I know there won't be a second and eating up an unnecessary chunk of my budget, among other things. Coffee has been my longest relationship, and while it had its dysfunctions - like making me have more seizures - we were happy. Boyfriends may have come and gone, but when I needed cheering up, I knew where to go. The open arms of lattes are always the right temperature: hot in the winter, iced in the summer. Fondness and sadness fill me with each memory.

Though still these days, no involuntary shaking since January, my hand feels empty. It feels the loss of a Dunn Brothers to-go cup, a Starbucks travel mug, a Colorado College Alumni ceramic coffee mug. There's a missing weight that leaves my hand empty, leaves my body wanting, leaves my mind uncaffeinated. I mourn the loss of an appendage I mercilessly hacked off with a machete and left to wither in a frozen gutter outside the Mayo Clinic.


**FM**


When I was fifteen, finally holding my learner's permit and looking at the driver's side door with a mixture of longing and fear, my dad took me driving. I hated driving. I was bad at it - really bad at it - and kept barely missing parked cars and pedestrians since every turn I made was either too wide or too narrow. It was exhausting! I knew it was a necessary evil and that one day I would be able to get in a car and drive around town without even thinking about it, but right then I was filled with self-doubt and loathing.

Every day he would pick me up from swim practice and ask, "Do you want to drive?"

I paused, knowing he wanted me to say yes, that I should say yes because I desperately needed the practice, but I could feel the anxiety already welling up inside of me. A rock wedged itself into the pit of my stomach and my chlorine-saturated armpits started to sweat. My heartbeat matched what it had clocked after a 50 yard sprint an hour ago. I wiped my clammy palms on the team-logoed sweatpants I'd pulled on over my wet swimsuit. I can do this. No, I can't. Yes, I can! No, I can't! I don't wanna and you can't make me!!

"No, dad, I'm good." My heart sank even as it slowed and I dropped my eyes as I tossed my bag, backpack and purse into the backseat and climbed into the front. I was relieved that I didn't have to perform the terrifying act that was dangerous to all parties involved and that made the thought of my Sweet Sixteen sour.

Last week, I started driving again for the first time since the surgery! This time, my anxiousness far outweighed my anxiety. My dad used to say that when he was a teenager, they called cars, "freedom machines", or "FM"s for short, and for the previous week, every time I had to ask for a ride and every time he drove me, I couldn't have agreed more. I love my dad, but despite his ability to get from point A to point B in a remarkably timely manner, I'm almost out of nausea pills.

Sunday night came, dark, cold and snowing lightly at four pm. I had choir and needed a ride. "Mom? Can you drive me to my rehearsal?"

"Sure, honey," she answered, not knowing what was in store for her.

I paused, feeling a little like Calvin from Calvin and Hobbs, slightly mischievous as I asked, "Can I drive?"

"Sure, honey," she replied, a bit slower this time, a small hint of knowledge that this might be a bad idea.

Excitement flooded me - at last, I could drive! Nine years after getting my drivers license, I really am a good driver and have never been in an accident with a car, a wayward pedestrian or a poorly-placed lamppost. My mom's hesitation was born of the fact that it had been just over a week ago that I was able to walk down staircases by myself and take a shower without requiring someone in the house to make sure I hadn't fallen if I was taking too long. Nonetheless, as we walked through the garage door and climbed in on sides that felt unfamiliar, each of us felt a flood of emotions that did not include calm or confident.

I turned the ignition and the car came to life, BBC on the radio (which she promptly turned off so it wouldn't split my focus) and a purring beneath me. A thrill ran through me, an electric current racing down my arms and legs. My foot found the break and held it down as I shifted to reverse and

186

looked behind me.

I took the longer way to my high school - the site of the rehearsal - keeping to main roads rather than the side streets I usually take, as smaller, residential streets hadn't been plowed and were still icy. I figured my cautious mom was nervous enough without her newly-driving daughter navigating a treacherous, poorly-lit route.

Yes, we made it safely to the school, and as I put the car in park in front of the newly-redone entrance, I could hear her mostly-internal sigh. We made it, was written across her face. A wave of fondness and gratitude for her patience washed over me.

I can drive. I am a driver. I am not broken. Most importantly, I'm cleared to re-claim my FM!


## Bills, Headaches and Haircuts

I can't believe this. I'm completely overwhelmed. And the best part is that it's all my fault that I'm screwed. I just feel awful about myself. What is wrong with me? Why did I miss that one payment? And then today I found out that J. Crew says I have a payment 60 days overdue, which has now affected my credit score, but I was never sent a bill! I feel like so much of my life right now is trying to figure this out, trying to fix my huge mistake, and I'm not even sure if it'll work. What if my appeal doesn't go through? What happens then? No other insurance carrier will take me because of my pre-existing condition. I don't have a job to get insurance through, and even if I can find a carrier or a plan, it's not going to start retroactively and pay for my surgery. COBRA will if my appeal is accepted. Please, God, let it be accepted. I can't handle this. I feel like a ridiculous, stupid, flaky, unreliable, irresponsible, failure. I just don't like myself these days. Sometimes I feel like I don't even respect myself. What happened?

The other night as I was carrying dinner plates covered in films of marinara sauce and small chunks of meatballs next to torn pieces of lettuce that couldn't stick to a fork, I said to my parents, "You know, sometimes lately I forget that I just had brain surgery." Despite my yo-yo rollercoaster mental health, physically I've been feeling pretty great. I've been active, getting out of the house almost every day, taking showers and doing my hair, writing, reading, not taking naps. As nice as it is to feel better, I forget that

I just had brain surgery, and have been pushing myself a little too much. Yesterday I paid the price for it, spending the majority of the day in bed with the worst headache I've had in weeks. My mind might have forgotten, but my body sure reminded it. I made it through probably six episodes of Lie To Me - one on the tv downstairs as I ate my Fruity Pebbles and the rest in bed after I decided that bed was a better idea than trying to function in the real world. Throughout the day, I took a few naps and more Tylenol, but no oxycodone. I thought about it, but opening the dark orange bottle and swallowing the little, white pill felt like too much of a step backward. Maybe that's silly, but it's what was going through my head.

Today I went out, all dressed up in a skirt and high-heeled boots, my hair shiny and crafted into perfect, light curls and waves. Adding a pearl necklace and silver earrings, I felt pretty, fashionable, classy. Tomorrow, I'm getting my hair cut. It will be a sad day. The long, dark brunette mane that still graces the right side of my head, neck and shoulder will be cut off and matched to its sister hemisphere: three-quarter inch spikes that grow in every direction. I made the appointment an hour ago, and part of me is regretting it already. I would've waited for another week, but Monday I go to Mayo for my follow-up appointments, one of which is an EEG, and getting the glue out of long hair takes days, while I'm guessing short hair is much easier to rid of gooey, blue chunks.

I woke up this morning with a headache, and though it's gone away, I think it would be wise to heed its warning and take a nap.

## Haircut

"I have to say, I'm a little nervous. I've never done this before." I handed my jacket to the hairdresser and stuffed my hat and scarf into my purse before setting it on the hair-covered floor with a wince and climbed into the chair. My heartbeat pounded in my ears as my eyes flitted back and forth between the long curls on one side of the Mississippi and the short spikes on the other.

I remembered my little sister's words from the day I told her that the doctors would have to shave half of my head: "Oh, Erica, my heart is breaking for you. If they told me that, I wouldn't do it." Needless to say, she's very attached to her hair, and right then, my heart was breaking for me, too.

188

The executioner held up a chunk of the long hair that I had crafted perfectly that morning for the last time, "Okay, this is going to look like a lot, but we have to get this out of the way before I shape it". I watched in horror as the scissors closed in, swimming at top speed through the air like Jaws toward a skinny dipping coed; I could hear the ominous theme song. Closer and closer they got until I could see the sharp teeth on their serrated blades. In slow motion, the scissors devoured the lock of hair, determined to be brave as it accepted its fate. I dropped my eyes, lacking the masochistic streak needed to watch.

The hairdresser stepped back, scissors hanging at ease from one finger, and lifted and pulled at different pieces in turn. "What do you think about doing something asymmetric?"

No, thanks. "Um, I'm not sure. What do you mean? I don't want something too..." I searched for another way to say unfortunate-looking 80's hipster, but came up empty, "yeah. I don't know."

He deliberated on my hair another minute before bringing the scissors to attention and digging in, cutting and shaping an asymmetrical creation. I watched with increasing skepticism, my fight or flight reflex kicking in when he started to snip at the hair on my left side that I'd been working so hard to grow out for the last two months. I bit back the, what the hell are you doing? and swallowed my anxiety. Suddenly he stopped, again stepping back and observing my head with the keen eye of a seasoned art critic. I looked in the mirror, trying to see what he saw, but all that stared back at me was half a head of super short hair and half a head of hair that reached half way down my ear. I waited for him to keep cutting, but he just looked at me, "What do you think?"

Bile rose in my throat as I realized that he intended to leave me this way, intended to let me walk out into the world looking like a sixteen year old boy whose friend had cut his hair in an act of parental defiance. "Yeah, I think this is too much for me," I attempted to deliver in a calm voice.

"So you want me to just make this side equal to that side?" he attempted to deliver in a calm voice, though I could hear the disappointment laced with disdain that dripped from it. Clearly I was quite less than cool; even straight up lame.

"Yeah," I replied a little sheepishly. Apparently "yeah" was the word of the day - a noncommittal way to begin a contradictory statement. As in, yeah, this is hideous, or, yeah, I know you think I'm a loser for it, but I really don't care and I want you to make my head even before I throw up. I've never been good at telling hairdressers that I didn't like what they did to me, but sometimes it's necessary, and I was proud of myself.

When he finished, my hair looking as vanilla as possible, I took a last look at myself and said a little prayer that I would still get hit on by more men than women before hopping off the chair. I had to admit that the cut was pretty cute. Not something I would've ever done on my own, but for a necessity cut, it wasn't bad at all.

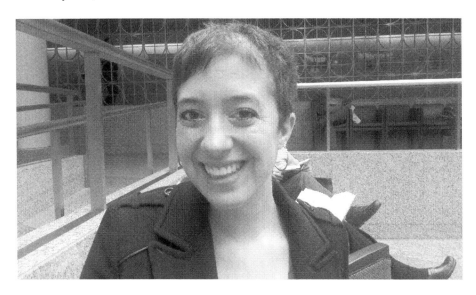

### Follow-Up Coming Up

Tomorrow I go to Mayo for the beginning of my follow-up testing. The alarm on my purple cell phone is set for 8:30am, giving me an hour and a half to shower, get dressed, make myself look presentable and have some breakfast before mom and I drive down to Rochester. The next three days and the following Monday will be tiring, stressful and full of nail biting.

Tomorrow is the neuropsych exam, the results of which I'm not worried about; I'm only thinking that I'll likely glaze over half way through it since it's a four hour exam, which is a much longer stretch of time than anything I've had to do since surgery. I'll bring a snack and it'll be fine, but last time I went, I got to bring a sixteen ounce latte with me.

190

Tuesday consists of the test I'm most worried about: the EEG. The MRI is on Tuesday as well, but the EEG is the test that will show if there's still seizure activity going on in my brain. The EEG will show us if the surgery was successful.

Wednesday I meet with the neurologist I've been working with at Mayo, and the following Monday, I see the neurosurgeon. Those days are when I'll get the results of the tests and have the chance to talk about options for my future. I haven't thought of questions to ask yet, but I'm working on it. If you have any ideas, please let me know.

I was talking to my mom tonight and she said that she's nervous to go back to Mayo because of all the feelings it will stir up as she walks the same halls she walked between the hospital cafeteria and my bedside. She asked me if I felt the same, but honestly, I don't. I think my surgeries were a traumatizing event for my parents, but a transformational one for me. Still, I'll let you know how we fare back in the Gonad - I mean Gonda - building.

## Parking Structures

I wasn't sure what I'd expected, but when we reached the streets of down-town Rochester, passing the hotel we stayed at the three nights before my first surgery and turned into the parking ramp opposite the Mayo and Gonda buildings, I felt nothing. No ghost of anxieties passed crept into the car to haunt me; my heart rate was steady and my breath deep and calm.

God love my mom, but she's the most nervous person I know when it comes to finding a parking spot. Up and up we spiraled, passing open spot after open spot, each one sufficiently wide and a perfectly fine candidate, but still we pressed on. The parking ramp switchbacks were starting to get to me, as was my mom's infuriating inability to just park already. I was nearing my wit's end when after passing three more open spots near the nineth floor elevator, she proceeded to the far end of the row and parked.

"Why did you do that? There were three perfectly good spots right by the door", I asked heatedly.

Her simple response: "Because I knew it would irritate you". She smiled and after a moment's deliberation, I laughed.

## Follow-Up Day One: Neuropsych

The elevator doors opened and the light next to the button marked "SL" switched off as we stepped into the subway level of the Mayo Clinic. A wave of nostalgia swept over me as I took in the silver block letters that spelled out "Gonda Building" above the streams of people coming and going like ants in an ant hill. The low-ceilinged hallway opened into a large, open atrium, the sound of a woman singing along with a piano echoing off the tall windows, grand staircase and hanging sculpture. I remembered it like I'd only been there yesterday, but my vivid recollection included just the building, not the testing and not the surgery, which still some days try to bury themselves in the sands of my mind like brightly colored coquinas on the beach.

My mom and I checked in and made our way to the first bank of elevators, a hanging sign in the Clinic's signature font noting it as service to floors eleven to eighteen. I pulled the folded itinerary out of my purse and double checked - 11:45am, Mayo Building, 11th floor West, Psychology. Today was to be a repeat of the neuropsych exam I had three days before the first surgery, just over two months ago.

The waiting room looked like any other: groupings of stiffly-padded chairs in various shades of mauve and hunter green spaced just far enough apart to allow for a degree of comfort and the option not to listen to another family's conversation while still being space-effective.

I sat down with the clipboard I'd been handed by the woman at the desk and began to check box after box after box with a no/yes ratio of about five to one. For the first time ever, I got to check yes for brain surgery under the "Have you had:" heading. I made my way through four pages of multiple choice questions, short answers and consent forms while a woman somewhere behind me coughed like there was no tomorrow. I made sure to saturate my hands and arms with antibacterial gel from the Costco-sized pump bottle at the front desk when I handed back my clipboard.

The neuropsych evaluation was an exact copy of the one I took two months ago while my skull was still fully intact and my body without titanium parts. For four hours, I listened to stories and lists of words and repeated them; ordered strings of numbers and letters before reciting them back to the proctor; viewed pictures for ten seconds and reproduced them from memory; found patterns in multi-colored cards; listed all of the

192

words starting with c as I could in one minute; gave descriptions of words, likely sounding quite pretentious as I did because of my uses of "which", "such" and myriad SAT vocabulary words; and finished with fifteen minutes of math.

At the three hour mark I was given a break to stretch my legs, drink my Snapple and check the emails on my phone, but when we left at four-o-clock I was exhausted. This was the longest I've had to concentrate since the last time I took the test, and the little stamina I had left took me straight to the cold room at the Marriott down the street and dumped me into bed. The covers left some to be desired; there seemed to be a thicker layer missing, but it didn't keep me from enjoying a two hour nap.

Tomorrow are the EEG and MRI, the results of which I'm looking forward to seeing, but I won't be given any until my appointment with the neurologist Wednesday and the neurosurgeon next Monday. Until then, there's no use in worrying, so all that's left is to watch Bones reruns on my ipod and fall asleep.


### Hot Cocoa
*7:30am, Tuesday, Day 2*

I watched as the hot cocoa mix clumped and floated on the surface of the hot water, brown bubbles with chunks sliding down them stuck to the side of the cup. I left the cup on the buffet while I searched for the little black stir straws that ended up being right under my nose.

The cocoa mix swirled and sank as I stirred, powder dispersing and dissolving in the water that was still too hot to drink. I grabbed a top and popped it onto the Styrofoam cup, first pressing down with my palm and then tracing the edge with my finger to be sure it was locked in place.

Dad carried my hot cocoa as I hefted my backpack and purse onto my shoulders and my overnight bag into the crook of my left arm. It had rained all through the night and a cold mist remained as we made our way to the car. I threw my bags in the back, climbed into shotgun and turned the seat heater on high.

Something in my eye was bothering me, so I flipped down the mirror to check it out; I found a clump of mascara floating there, a sailor overboard from the ridge of my lower right lid. I stuck my finger in my eye the way that used to gross me out as a kid when I saw grownups do it, and wondered, not for the first time this morning, why I'd bothered to wear make-up when I was about to get glue in my hair and wasn't even planning to see anyone I knew. Force of habit, I guess. I had a feeling that if I had long hair, I would've skipped it.

We pulled into the parking ramp with 20 minutes to go, and got in line for the elevator that would take us to the subway level, from which we could reach the next elevator bank to the seventh floor of the Gonda building - Neuro.

Dad waited behind me while I checked in at the EEG desk. I was told they'd call my name when they were ready for me, so we walked through the maze of chairs to an empty section in the back where we could set our drinks on a side table and split the newspaper after I turned my phone on silent.

A woman in dark blue scrubs called my name over the speaker, surprising me by pronouncing it correctly. Leaving my bulk of coat and scarf with my dad, I walked down the one straight aisle amid the waiting room chairs.

The EEG tech escorted me over the threshold that separates the patients from the people who hold their hands. She chatted as we walked down the echoing hallway with its linoleum floor, turning this way and that, each door we passed eliciting a, "Just a little bit farther!".

Just a little bit farther, we came to a room with two chairs: a green one for my coat and purse and a black one for me. As I sat, my hat stuffed in my bag, the tech draped a hospital gown over my back and shoulders to protect my zip up sweatshirt from the glue. I let her know that the left side of my head was still pretty tender but for the spot toward the top that's numb. I said I was okay with having a little numb spot on my head after everything else had turned out perfectly.

For the next thirty minutes, we talked about life, families, sisters, nieces, nephews and grandchildren. She was as careful as she could be as she applied the electrodes to my head, but it still hurt. I almost asked her to hand me my Tylenol from my purse, but figured I'd wait 'til the test was done.

With a little help, I got up from the chair and walked to a room with a bed next door, she following behind me, carrying the leads that had been so diligently applied.

I sat in a chair by the bed for the first part of the test: seeing my brain functioning. I looked at pictures, read out loud, hyperventilated for three minutes and looked into a strobe light as it grew faster and faster. Finally the pounding light stopped and I was told to lie down on the bed and sleep for half an hour so they could get a baseline. Sleep? Music to my ears! I all but leaped into bed and snuggled under the blankets she laid on top of me. In less than two minutes, I was fast asleep. (Ah but to be asleep right now! Alas, I'm waiting in the lobby for my ride.)

Half an hour later I was awoken, and retuning to my chair, the tech took the leads and stickers off my head and gently rubbed out most of the glue with something that smelled like nail polish remover and made me cough when I inhaled it.

Dad wasn't in the waiting room where I'd left him, but both of our coats were... The phone rang three times as I held it to my ear before, "Hello!"

"Where are you, dad? I just got out."

"Oh! About a hundred feet away. You can probably see the gray back of my head if you turn around."

I looked around, sweeping the ocean of chairs, all littered with gray backs of heads, before he stood up, turned around and waved at me. A smile spread across my face; what was he doing over there and why did it seem like a good idea to leave our stuff behind? I gave up trying to understand his lack of common sense long ago.

As he walked over, I offered, "Wanna get some lunch?"


## Day Of Reckoning Eve

Last night I stayed in a cold hotel room a five minute car ride from the Clinic. When I woke up with a kink in my neck, it only made sense that I was going to a day of hospital tests. Tonight I'm back home, watching yesterday's new episode of Castle on the DVR in the living room, after which I get to go up to my own bed. But tomorrow I have to go back down to Mayo; and this time it's not for tests. The sweet smell of flowers in my room, the rain on the window panes, they lull me into a false sense of safety, of on-the-other-sidedness, because tomorrow is not just another lovely day in the neighborhood; tomorrow is the Day of Reckoning.

At one pm, I will go in and meet with the neurologist I've been working with at Mayo, and he'll tell me the results of the tests I took yesterday and today. All three neuropsych, EEG and MRI were standard and passed uneventfully, but the results will tell us if the surgeries were successful. The EEG is really the one I'm anxious about, since it's the one that shows if there's still any seizure activity left in my brain.

My head hurts from having electrodes glued on and taken off of it, being compressed with foam to keep it still during the MRI and finally from me picking glue chunks out of my hair. A couple leads went on my scar, as it travels down a good length of the middle of my head, where a few electrodes needed to go. Those have been particularly difficult to get glue off of because the picking, scratching and tugging really irritate the seam holding me together and the traumatized scalp around it.

Since the day I decided to have this surgery back in October, it's never really occurred to me that it might not be successful. Obviously I knew it was a possibility, a fairly large one, at that, but deep down, I always assumed that no matter what, no matter the odds, of course it would work. Now I don't know.

The past week or so, I've occasionally gotten a light or weak sensation in my right hand, and it kind of reminds me of a watered-down version of the feeling I used to get during a seizure. Maybe I'm just making it up, my peppy, positive imagination doubting itself and running the other way, or maybe it's just a remnant of the functionality and sensation I lost when the resection was completed. My sister reminded me today that even if it turns out to be seizure activity, the doctors did say that in the first couple months, it's not uncommon to have a couple seizures as your body figures out what the hell you just did to it, which did help calm the funnel cloud of thoughts in my mind and lift the growing weight on my chest. Clearly it wouldn't be ideal, but the fact remains that I've been seizure-free for two months. Even if there is seizure activity left, my epilepsy has improved dramatically. That's my chin up talking, and I'll hold on to any silver lining I can get my hands on until my knuckles are white.

196

## Snow Check

Well, we've gotten about six inches of snow so far, sitting atop a layer of ice, and it's still coming down, so we've decided to take a "snow check". Driving conditions are far from safe, so at the behest of my parents, I called the Mayo neurologist's office and asked to reschedule. I haven't heard back yet on the new time/date, but should in the next hour or so.

I have to say that I'm pretty disappointed. I've been mentally preparing for this meeting and I really want the results of my tests. This morning as I was putting on my eyeliner, my hand felt strange, and it scared me. I don't know if it was a seizure or if I'm imagining things. I hate the fears and uncertainties going on in my head, the thoughts spinning around and around wondering if maybe this didn't work. I just want answers. That's all. I want to know if there's still seizure activity in my brain. This limbo is draining me. I'm remembering what it felt like back in November and December, being paralyzed by the unknown.

A thought flitted into my head, just for a moment, asking what there is in my life that I can control, and my automatic response was food. If there had been a mirror before me, I would have seen my face contort in disgust at my answer. I'm glad that that was my reaction. It's comforting to know.

When we decided definitively not to drive to Rochester, I could feel my mom seeing the disappointment in me and how sad it made her to watch me. Being a mom, she's good at sensing those things and knowing how to fix them. Maybe it's not a cure, but certainly to dampen the symptoms, she suggested that we walk to the diner a few blocks away and have breakfast. I intend to get something greasy and unhealthy that will taste amazing going down but will probably make me feel sick the rest of the day. I'm okay with that.


## Lip Zits

I have a zit on my face. A really blatant one, right on my upper lip, taunting me. Lip zits are by far the most painful to pop. I mean exceedingly painful, but I was determined. Leaning forward to see it better, I placed one fingernail on each side and pressed through the pain until a chunk of white puss shot out and landed on the mirror. I kept going, wanting to make sure there was nothing left in the raised hole I'd created, and pretty sure there was, but I was unable to get it.

When I got out of the shower, the zit's ground zero hole was still all red and surrounded by pink. It needed to be hidden. I tried to put heavy-duty concealer on it, layer foundation over that and then top it off with some setting powder, but when I stepped back from the mirror, it just laughed at me. The red was covered - for the time, at least - but the bump of it stuck out so far that it caught light from the lamp across the room and cast its own shadow over my Chapsticked lips. I had been defeated.

In the past week, I've broken out on my face, my chest and my back. It's gross. What's bothering me is that back zits have a nickname: bacne (pron: back-nee, like acne), but chest zits are totally left out. No nickname for the little red bumps that preclude me from wearing most of my shirts as I have an affinity for scoop necks.

Wednesday I was supposed to go back to Mayo and see my neurologist, who would tell me the results of the tests I'd had the two days before. Wednesday I was supposed to find out if there's still seizure activity in my brain or not. Wednesday, seven inches of snow covered a layer of ice that spanned the width and length of every street and highway in town. And out of town, for that matter. We had planned to leave the house at ten, giving us plenty of time to get to the one-o-clock appointment since it's only an hour and a half drive to Rochester, but the snow was still falling, thick, white flakes dancing quickly through the air. The tv said that the storm was moving South, toward Rochester. The driving conditions were growing more dangerous by the minute; it would be crazy to attempt a trip to Mayo.

I called the neurology office to see if I could reschedule my appointment for Monday, when I was planning to come down to see the surgeon. Would that be okay? Did he have any openings? I was so disappointed. I wanted so badly to see the results of those tests, to know if the surgeries worked, to know what was happening in my body. I had mentally prepared myself for whatever answer I would get; or at least prepared myself not to fall to the ground crying with either grief or gratitude. But no, that would be another day. I had all of this energy and emotion stored up and ready to go but nowhere to use it. The adrenaline evaporated, leaving me sapped, disappointed and angry. I so rarely get angry; I hate that feeling. I was angry at the snow, at the ice, at the world for keeping me scared and anxious.

The office called back at about eleven with a new time for my appointment, which they were able to get on Monday. The negative emotions inside of me were exhausting, but I mustered up a genuine thank you for all of her help.

I spent a lot of the day sleeping, reading and watching Hulu on my computer, and by dinner I was okay. I'd accepted that I was going to have a few more days of uncertainty. I knew I would be scared and impatient, but I learned how to deal with that in the months before the surgeries and I could do it again. So now I wait.

Since middle school, I've learned that stress has a funny (not ha ha funny) way of bringing friends with it, most of whom cause their own stresses. Specifically, I'm referring to zits. Lots of 'em. I hoped that they would go away once I heard definitively if there was any seizure activity still in my brain, but now I have three more days for my body to express how it feels about being in limbo by turning me into Pizza Face.

Wait, there's another undergrounder surfacing on my lip... ugh.


**Love Cocoon**

"Listen, there's no traffic on the lake", mom noted.

It's that in between time where the ice is too thin for trucks, ice houses, snowmobiles or pedestrians, but the lake isn't open enough for boats or jetskis. Swimmers won't venture in until late May, and even then they'll be in wetsuits til June.

Mom and I sat at the near end of the long, wooden table whose leaf was still in from the fundraiser we hosted last weekend. The rhythmic whoosh of the dishwasher played backup to Corinne Baily Rae as we contemplated the everything and nothing of life between conversations. Dad had already left to watch basketball in their bedroom, but the dampened sound of an announcer punctuated by shoes screeching on the court let us know that he was still nearby.

At dinner, after discussing Elizabeth Taylor, Marilyn Monroe, and the twenty first century paparazzi's role in the death of the untouchable Hollywood star, and before going over the HBO specials mom wants me to set up on the dvr when we get back in town, the three of us put together a list of questions to ask the doctors on Monday. As they each gave their opinions on what to add to the list I'd already written or how to re-word what I'd said, I managed to only interrupt to contradict two or three times and didn't roll my eyes once! I'm learning patience and calm.

I've learned a lot since moving back home; I can't believe it's almost time for me to leave. This is likely my last night at the cabin. Of course, my parents remind me every other day that I could stay and can live with them as long as I want, and that the cabin is empty all week and I could stay there if I wanted space, and every time the topic of my move date comes up, mom says that we should wait and see how I feel when we get back from our upcoming Big Sigh of Relief trip to the Bahamas. I don't know if there's ever going to be a perfect time to move back to Denver; I just have to leap and have faith that I'll land without spraining an ankle. It's gonna be hard leaving my little love cocoon here, but the time is coming for me to break into a butterfly and fly away. A butterfly with a big, bold stripe down the middle of its back.

The image of a butterfly floated through the everything and nothing in my mind, and I answered, "I know, it's nice."


**Recording**

The past week or so, I've been writing down my memories of the hospital, the surgeries, each one a vignette caught in type like a firefly on fly paper. I sift through the foggy recesses of my mind, drug- and pain-induced clouds concealing the whole picture but letting one memory at a time float to the surface like the answer in a Magic 8 Ball. The scene is revealed to me and suddenly I'm right back there, lying in bed, my thoughts oscillating between the present and the future, fear and excitement.

I want to write, I want to record everything I felt, saw, smelled, touched, pin it down before it fades away, but it's not easy. I shake the Magic 8 Ball of my mind and a memory floats up in response, and as promised, I can see, feel and smell, but what I find is not always good. So many things there were easier when I didn't know what was coming. I waltzed blithely (or more likely crawled blindly) through each decision, toward each procedure, knowing nothing about the fear and pain that waited on the other side. That made it easier at the time, but now when I go back, the fear and the pain stick out. I don't like remembering those parts.

When I put myself back there, looking through my same eyes, the strong, courageous heroine I'm proud of now is a scared little girl whose head hurts so much she can hardly move.

It's hard to remember those things, it really is, but I need to record them. I force myself back there and I write down as much as I can, because even if no one else ever reads it, I want my children to know what their mom did for them. I want them to know the strength inside themselves and believe that they can trust it.

## Follow-Up w Surgeon

I'm at Mayo for my last day of follow-ups: seeing my doctors to get the results of my tests last week. I just saw my surgeon and got amazing news: they didn't find any seizure activity left in my brain!! This is the news I've been praying for - it couldn't be any better. More to come, but thank you all from the bottom of my heart for your prayers and good wishes!


Erica Egge
I've got a clean head! No seizure activity!! Yahoo!!!

Chris, Charlie, Thomas and 46 others like this.

Sarah Awesome little cousin! Simply awesome!
Chuck Congrats Erica!
Keri That's such good news. Cause for celebration!!!
Natalie YAY Erica!!!
Stacy YAY!!!! Now come home!!
Megs Yay!!!!! Love ya!
Erica Egge Thanks, guys! I'm pretty darn excited myself!
Catherine So, so happy to hear you are doing well. However you are still in my daily prayers. Love you. Your Uncle Pete's favorite mother-in-law
Katie So thrilled!!
Anna Congratulations! that is so amazing
Merima Wahooo!
Madeline YES!! Amazing Erica! :)
Eve I am SO SO SO SO SO SO SO SO SO HAPPY!!!!!!!!!!!!!!!! AHHH-

HHHH!!!!!!!!!!!!!!!!!
Kevin EGGE! thats amazing! im really happy for you right now!
Neil !!!!!!!!!!!!!!!!!!!!!!!!!!!!!!
Hannah Congratulations! think of all that free space...
Erin Yay!!!!!!
Catherine Do you realize how fortunate you are YOU HAVE SO MANY
FRIENDS WHO LOVE YOU. INCLUDING ME.
Kyle That's great news Erica!!
Erica Egge Thank you guys! You're making me tear up a little... :)
Catherine Think of you daily


## It Hardly Feels Real

I still can't believe it. I'm seizure-free. The doctors were clear that a clean
EEG didn't mean I was cured, but it's a good sign. A really good sign.
There is no abnormal, epilepgenic activity in my brain. The doctors also
talked about the pathology report on the chunk of brain that they took out.
Apparently it was a cortical dysplasia that had bothered me for so many
years. What that means is that when my little fetus brain was forming,
a few neurons missed the train and ended up growing in some incorrect
fashion, forming what we've been calling "The Birthmark", and causing
me to have seizures. And now I'm quite sure The Birthmark is lying in a
biohazard bag in the back of a truck headed toward biowaste heaven.

Wow. I mean, really, wow. I can't get over it. I never thought this day
would come; never truly thought it possible. The neurologist said that in
July, as long as I'm still seizure-free, I can start to wean off one of my
three seizure meds, and if I'm still clean next January, a year from the surgery, I can get off another one! He says I'll more than likely always be on
at least a small dose of one medication, just to be safe, but that's fine. In
the mean time, though, I have good news and bad news: the good news is
that I can drink decaf again! He thinks that coffee won't end up being any
kind of problem, but to start slow and keep it at decaf for now. The bad
news: no drinking for a year. A YEAR! I was hoping to have a little some-
thin'-somethin' to celebrate tonight, but I guess that'll have to be sparkling
lemonade in a martini glass. Bummer, but again, I'm okay with that. One
year alcohol-free for a lifetime seizure-free? No contest.

"Wow", "phew", "wahoo!" and similars are the only things I've been able
to say to express this... this whatever-it-is, wordless phenomenon. It hasn't

202

sunk in yet. I have a new life. Like, seriously, a new life. It hardly feels real, but somehow, magically, it is.

**God,**

Thank you. Thank you for Your blessings. Thank you for giving me what could become a whole new life. I am so grateful to You. None of this really feels real yet. I feel like this is one of the biggest days of my life so far and I'm not savoring it the way I should. I don't really know how I feel right now, maybe a little confused and grasping as the last bit of the day slips away before I can figure it out. God, please help me to sort out my feelings. Please help me to accept the end of my seizures, which have defined me and set me as other for my whole life, and help me to accept and understand that my surgery worked, that I don't have seizures anymore! Thank you.

I'm a little scared that I'll end up like that lady who wrote that she was seizure-free for fourteen months before her seizures came back a lot worse than they'd ever been. Please, please don't let that happen to me. That would be so awful, so heartbreaking. I don't think I could do this surgery again. Rather, I could with Your love behind me, but it would be so much harder. But this news is indeed good.

Please look over my family. Please make sure they know how incredibly much I love them and let them sleep well tonight.

All this I pray in Your holy name,

Amen.

**Packing Tired Cobras**

It's my second to last night here before I move back to Colorado. I'm sitting cross-legged under the yellow striped duvet that covers my bed. The left side of the bed is covered with scarves and t-shirts that still have to be packed and two legal pads that I need to find a home for. This morning dad and I picked up some cardboard boxes I found free on Craig's List - three long, skinny boxes with handles, two big boxes and one small square one. I won't need all of them, but as I put everything together, I'm surprised at how much stuff I need to get back to Colorado. Since I'll be back here a couple times over the next few months for weddings and doctor appointments, I'll be able to collect and bring back whatever I leave here, so right now I'm only taking about half of my things. Still, half is turning out to take up more space than I would've guessed. They're all things I've used though, not just superfluous junk, which makes me feel better.

Today I found out that COBRA has decided to reinstate me. I can't begin to say how amazing I feel. A current of nervous electricity ran through me as I opened the email and read, "Hi Erica, I got you approval for reinstatement". An enormous weight was lifted off of my Atlas shoulders. I started laughing in my car, parked in front of my therapist's office, looking, I'm sure, like a total nut job, not quite sure if I should welcome or blink back the tears that waited just behind my eyes. I picked my phone back up and my hands shook as I typed my reply on the little slide-out keyboard. Everything has gone so much better than I could have ever hoped - the surgeries, the follow-up, the insurance - everything. I guess I must've done something right!

I feel like there are so many things I want to write about, so many little experiences, feelings, thoughts that I want to word, like a river inside me that transforms into a sparkling, sunkissed waterfall as it leaves my mouth and flows onto the page. I want to write about packing and the conflicting emotions it brings, knowing that it's the right time for me to go but already missing my parents and my aunts; how I can look in a mirror and like what I see and not feel all of the insecurities I felt in the Bahamas; how I started to use my body again as I walked to the Sea Center (or whatever it's called) in the Bahamas for nine am yoga, and how I almost passed out more than once during that first class but every day got better and better as the young instructor taught patiently in both English and French ("inspirer, expirer" = "breathe in, breathe out"). I want to write about them all, but not tonight. My heavy eyelids are drooping over the eyes I got peach-scented soap in when I washed my face this evening, which I take as my cue to go to sleep.

Goodnight

### Goodbye Prelude to a Shower

At seven am, Remix To Ignition started to fill the silence covering my bedroom. Starting quietly, it grew and grew, like a weed with tentacles that reached out with a crescendo. I stirred, sleep fading from my eyes, dripping down to be absorbed again by my bed. I rolled onto my back and began to mouth along the lyrics, adding improvised hand motions to illustrate the words being sung ("Give me that toot toot, give me that beep beep" eliciting a train whistle and a honking horn).

When the song was over, I slid the "Off" button and climbed out of bed. I had more packing to do, but first, a shower. Mom and dad's shower is nice and big and roomy compared to mine – both mine in the house and mine in my apartment – so obviously I wanted to use theirs for my Last Shower. I grabbed my towel and padded down the hallway in ripped plaid pajama pants and a t-shirt that advertised my milkshake as bringing all the boys to the yard. I crossed the familiar threshold into my parents' room, the room I'd crept into countless times in the middle of the night as a child. This morning I felt like a child again, missing my parents already.

"Can I use your shower or do you need it?"

My mom looked at me, makeup done, wearing a black suit skirt under a pajama top, her hair still damp. Dad sat in bed with a cup of coffee and the Journal. Mom's eyes had the glass and the sad, proud, conflicted smile that only a parent can wear. She stepped forward and hugged me to her, both of us trying not to cry. "I've loved having you here. I'm gonna miss having you around." Her arms stayed around me, no intention of letting go. "You've really taken your place in this family, and I hope you hold onto it. We're gonna make sure you do."

I've thought about that many times, wishing hard that the three of us hold on to the closeness we've found and being nervous that we'll lose it. "I love you so much and I'm so proud of you." The mom look of love threatened to pull tears from my eyes when she stepped back and held me by the shoulders. She went on about how proud she is of me and how much she loves me and all of the other things I try to hold on to and remember so that one day I can treasure them when she's gone. Even writing about it makes me sad.

Her hair was still damp as she instructed me to call her every day. One more kiss and I turned around the way I'd come to wash up in a shower the size of my whole bathroom.

# Epilogue

The blue glue has formed dry clumps that stick to my scalp and cling to the base of each hair springing forth from it. I must say, though, that getting it out this time is much easier than when I had long hair. I turn the pink bottle of Garnier Fructis conditioner upside down and watch a long, creamy snake emerge and coil onto my palm. I run my hands through my hair, feeling rough spots where the EEG leads had been this morning. The tech who put them on suggested putting conditioner in dry hair and letting it sit for a bit before combing out the glue and rinsing. I turn the black dial on the wall of my parents' bathroom and shut the sliding glass doors of the shower as it fills with steam. I figure fifteen minutes will be enough time: five minutes to fill with white fog and ten to saturate my dry skin and coughing lungs. The steam swallows me as I step into the tan tile enclosure, sliding the warped and frosted glass behind me. I stand with my back to the tap, letting the hot air warm my body. I have to inhale slowly through my nose to avoid the water-induced coughing that feels like choking. I let my muscles relax and melt for a bit; it has been a long day.

My alarm went off at five thirty, Maroon 5 cutting through the early morning silence in the Rochester Garden Hilton. My mom stirred next to me as if she'd already been awake a few moments; John (my boyfriend of nine months and friend of two years) tried to sleep through it but I could see him twitch from his bed a few feet away. We brushed our teeth and washed our faces and my mom and I put on a little make up though it didn't do much to hide the bags under our eyes. In fifteen minutes, we were dressed, packed and out the door. The air outside was cold, a stark contrast from the desert climate of our room. Fortunately the car wasn't far away and it felt like no more than a minute had passed when we pulled into the best parking spot I'd had yet at the Mayo Clinic.

Gently I inhale, my hand covering my nose and mouth to shield my lungs from the saturated air of the shower-turned-steam-room. No water runs, just a stream of steam spitting out from a small, silver spigot four inches below the faucet. I stand, turn, pace on the tile floor of the tub, the movement and my thoughts keeping me company as I wait for the conditioner to do its magic.

When we arrived at the door, the Gonda building was locked. "The doors don't open til six thirty," said a guard. A handful of other early arrivals sat

208

on chairs or leaned against the glass wall separating the heated inter-door-way space from the white marble atrium.

"What time is it, mom?" I asked.

"Six ten," she replied. "Let's go get some breakfast." Caribou Coffee stood with warm welcoming arms across the street and down the block. I had oatmeal, John had a breakfast sandwich and mom had a coffee. I grabbed a paper napkin printed with the Caribou logo and a short holiday-themed Mad Lib. We ate our food and conversed in a series of requested adjectives and nouns, which I entered onto the napkin using the pen I lifted from our hotel room. The result was a mildly amusing story of buying bacon presents for your scissors and decorating a Christmas chair.

Our spirits lightened noticeably with food in our stomachs and we headed back to the hospital, checking in and being directed to the elevators to the desk on the eight floor of the Mayo building.

I'm quite convinced that the elevator in the Mayo building is the slowest in the continental U.S. It rose oh so incredibly slowly and steadily until the climbing light illuminated a black, printed "8", eliciting a ding and a slight lurch as the doors slid open. We stepped out into an unlit elevator bank, a little concerned as we turned the corner to find an empty room facing an empty check-in desk with half of its lights still out. We took a seat in three adjacent chairs upholstered in a familiar mauve floral pattern and waited.

Standing in the steam, I pick up the pink comb on the ledge next to me and begin running it through my hair; first one direction, then the next. I push the teeth along my scalp just above the hair line; I comb left, picking up glue and wiping it onto my leg, then comb right, finding a little more, and last forward, leaving wet hair hanging straight over my forehead like bangs with a slight curl at the edge where it meets my eyes.

We must have waited for fifteen minutes for the first person to open the desk for business. I checked in and sat back down, watching the clock between turns at Scrabble on my mom's iPad for another thirty. My EEG was set to begin at seven thirty, but as seven thirty came and went, I returned to the front to make sure we were in the right place. We weren't. "We're on the other side of the elevators," I reported, my voice full of urgency and tinged with fear.

"We'll grab your stuff, you run over there," mom replied with a rustle of nylon-blend jackets stuffed with down.

I all but sprinted to the desk at the far end of the long hallway, my support team in tow. "Hi," I panted, "I'm Erica," loud inhale, loud exhale, "I have an EEG at seven thirty."

"Okay, I'll let them know you're here."

Mom and John had settled in chairs that formed a corner around a light wooden end table. I sighed with relief that I hadn't missed it altogether. "Do you have to go to the bathroom, honey? You're gonna be in there for awhile."

With the exasperated look only a daughter can give her mother, I replied, "I do now." My previously undemanding bladder suddenly craved a door emblazoned with a stick figure in a dress under a sign reading, "Women." "Do I have time?" I asked, my eyes searching frantically.

"You'll be fine. I'll tell them you'll be right back." The believable assurance only a mother can give her daughter.


The glue comes out almost easily with each scrape of the comb. I run my fingers through my hair every couple minutes to find the next shadow of an electrode. My hands and arms have become covered with dark, almost black, hair and little rubbery balls of glue. The steam has stopped its flow and I reach for the silver handle on the wall, pulling it upward to start a stream of hot water from the bath faucet. I rinse my hands and the comb in the falling stream and watched the discarded clumps travel down the drain before carefully placing the white, rubber plug.


A tech in scrubs led me through the Authorized Personnel Only door and down the hallway to a make-shift room blocked from the world by a curtain on a curved metal ceiling track. "Hi, I'm," I forget her name, so I'll call her Morgan, "Morgan. How are you?"

We made friendly small talk about Denver, Minnesota, my boyfriend,

210

her husband, the weather, etc., while she dotted my head with pen, marking where the electrodes would go. After it was checked by her boss and revisions were made, Morgan began affixing each of about twenty seven electrodes to my scalp. "I remember the paste they used to use when I was a kid," I recounted, "It took forever to get out. I would inevitably miss some and it would flake to my shoulders for a week, looking like really big, gross dandruff."

She laughed, "Yeah, that's what I always hear. The glue is much better than the paste." It seemed to take forever to get each one placed and stuck in securely, but I was enjoying the company. Two double-checkings by the superior in a white coat and I was ready to go.

My favorite part about EEGs is nap time. I'm almost always tired and am very good at napping, especially when I didn't sleep well the night before and had to get up early. I laid down in the plastic bed and was covered with two blankets, heavy in weight but strangely not in thickness. The lights were turned off and it was time to start.

I watch as clear water pours from the faucet. It splashes cold on my feet and I push aside the drain plug with my toes, keeping my hand under the flow until it turns warm and I replace the white rubber. It fills quickly at first, rising a few inches before the change in depth becomes less noticeable, like a child aging - growing and morphing a little slower each time you visit until one year he looks the same as the last and the progress is visible only over three years, then five, then ten.

I sit on the floor, obstructing the tide that flowed from the origin to the farthest reaches. The sweat that sticks to me in the aftermath of the steam washes away, but though I am grateful to feel it leave, I can only think of how dirty the floor of a shower is. My mom used to call baths butt soup. She's right. Bubbles, "bath bombs" and gels fail to mention their real purpose as a mask that makes you forget you're simply stewing in your own filth. However, a bath tends to save water and heat when you plan to stay for another forty minutes to pull and pick clump after clump of glue out of your hair.

As much as I love the napping aspect of an EEG, I hate the parts that try to induce a seizure: strobe lights and hyperventilation. Moving from the bed to a chair, I heard the words I most hate: "Okay, I want you to breathe in and out a lot harder and faster than you normally would." It was a nice way of saying, "sit quiet and still but breathe like you're in the finishing stages of a marathon." Reluctantly I complied, knowing that though it would be three of the longest minutes of my day, it was only three minutes. Silly me, I always forget that it's not really three minutes. They say it is, but I swear it's got to be at least thirty. "Okay," Morgan said an eternity later in her most encouraging voice, "you're half-way through." *Are you kidding me?* was all I could think.

Finally, "Alright, you can breathe normally again." Thank God. "How do you feel?"

"Gross. Light headed and a little nauseous."

"That's normal."

No, really? I never would have guessed, was the snarky response in my head.

Next up: strobe lights. The room switched back into darkness and a large light was positioned directly in front of my face. This is meant to trigger seizures in photo-sensitive epileptics. The light flashed, so bright, less than a foot from my eyes. One flash. Another flash. A third. It started slowly. Every thirty seconds or so, it paused for just a moment and I heard a, "good job. You're doing great," before it started again, faster each time. Flash, flash, flash. Pause. Flash flash flash. Pause. Flashflashflashflash-flashflash. My eyes watered and I felt pain all the way through them. Erica, you can do this, I told myself. You've done this before. Be strong. Keep your eyes open.

In time, another series started, this time with my eyes closed. It was less unpleasant, though not much.

When the strobe stopped and the gentle overhead lights came on, all I had left were the easy things: blinking, reading and looking at a picture. I sat in the plastic chair and was asked to close my eyes. Stay awake, but close my eyes. Fat chance. I fell asleep almost immediately. They took turns coming into the room and rustling papers, tapping their feet to keep me awake. I tried to focus on the sounds they made, but fell asleep over and over despite myself.

Removing the electrodes was much quicker than placing them, but the solution that dissolved the glue smelled like nail polish remover being poured over my head. I said goodbye to Morgan and went back to the waiting room to find that I'd been gone for three hours.

Blue flecks float on the water, making circles around each other and around me. A couple times I drain some of the room temperature soup to make room for fresh hot water. I arch my back, reaching my hair to the bath's wet surface to rinse out what I can. The dark brown strands are soft from the handfuls of conditioner and I slowly sweep my head from side to side, feeling the water move between them. Comb, dip, comb, dip, punctuated with the occasional application of more pink cream, and slowly but surely I make progress.

We had some time before the appointment with my neurologist, so we made our way to the lab to get my blood drawn before a lunch of bagel sandwich and juice. My hair was still sticky and smelly, but it felt good to get some food in me.

Dr. S's office is back on the eighth floor and we took our time returning to the desk where we'd started our day. Not sure if the woman there recognized me, I approached her with a self-conscious, "Hi... I have an appointment with Dr. S... I was here earlier."

A flicker of possible recognition: "Oh, yeah, welcome back." She watched the monitor below the desk as the click of keys floated over the partition. "Here," she handed me a plastic pager like the kind seen at Applebee's, "When this goes off, go over to that door there."

A red light blinked and the pager vibrated, commanding attention while we gathered up our coats and bags. Another woman in blue scrubs led us down the hallway to an exam room. "The doctor will be right in." Mom, John and I looked at each other and I grabbed out the green notebook that's accompanied me every day like a security blanket since May of 2009. I flipped through pages of wedding toasts, insurance information, dates for MRIs, EEGs, appointments, my Mayo patient number, which I could have recited by heart, notes on companies in both Denver and Minneapolis that might possibly hire me, finally settling on the list of questions for Dr. S that we'd come up with the night before:

Still having headaches - is that normal? What could be causing it? What should I do?

When can I start to be active again - riding bikes, skiing, etc. - assuming it doesn't hurt me?

When can I drink alcohol and caffeine again?

What was the thing I had last week when my hand was acting funny? It didn't move like it would when I had a seizure, but it had a similar sensation...

The door opened and Dr. S walked in, white coat billowing slightly behind him. Our three-person party stood to shake his hand like a reception line at a wedding, or a funeral, or a graduation. Seats were resumed and the usual niceties were exchanged. "How are you feeling?" started the session and I started in on my list.

No, headaches are not normal at this stage. We'll have you get a CT.

You shouldn't start until we know what's causing the headaches.

Wait on alcohol and caffeine until we've gotten you off of the Vimpat and you're just on the Lamictal XR.

Hmm...

The last question was the one I was afraid to ask; the one I would have avoided if the contingent of Team Erica hadn't been in the room with me. Please, God, I prayed, don't let it be a seizure. He wasn't sure. My EEG from that morning showed no seizure activity, so it could have been psychosomatic - my body remembering the feeling of a seizure without actually having one. On the other hand, it could have been a small seizure.

"Just to be safe, let's increase your Lamictal a bit." Damn. I had been so looking forward to decreasing my medications, not adding more. The Lamictal has always given me dreadful side effects, which is why I took it only at night. I had no desire to go back to the dizziness, nausea and double vision that used to punctuate my mornings.

He reminded me that there was no seizure activity in my brain, so it was likely not an actual seizure. I clung to that as if my life depended on it. It couldn't have been one; the EEG showed that. The mantra continues like a marquee behind my eyes.

The rest of the visit passed uneventfully, walking in a straight line, walk-

ing on my toes then heels, touching my nose and touching his finger, pointing to the hand whose fingers wiggled. Dr. S had seen an article on me and my blog in the Epilepsy Foundation of Minnesota's newsletter and asked if I would mind sending him the picture of me from it for him to use in a presentation on my surgery to a neurology group in Venezuela. My name would be changed, of course, but they like to have a face to put to the story. I didn't care if he used my real name, but apparently it's protocol. "Sure, I'll send it over," I promised and he handed me a card with his email address.

Again, we all stood and shook his hand in turns and he left with well-wishes and an order for a CT scan.

John sat in the front seat as mom drove home, chatting about the visit, NPR and life as I dozed in the back, my head resting against the seat belt, heavy eyelids drooping over a scene of frozen corn fields.


A funnel forms like a tornado as the bath water drains through the hole in the tiled floor. I pull the handle for the shower on my way to standing and a sheet of water hits my back, trickling down my legs, rinsing away the soap scum left by the stagnant water of the bath. I wonder as I run a luffa over my body what the CT will show. Would it be more fluid built up? If so, how would they fix it? Would they have to go back in with a burr hole and a syringe to suck it out? How long would that recovery be? Obviously not nearly as long, but still, another surgery? When is this going to end? What about my hair? It's taken me a YEAR to grow it from peach fuzz to the tight curls that hang a couple inches below my earlobes. I know, it's just hair, but still! It's one of many symbols of how far I've come. Could they give me some kind of pill to dry me out instead? Might it drain itself over time?

I turn off the shower and listen to the last of the water rush through the pipes in the wall as I slide open the glass door and grab an over-sized cream-colored towel, patting down my body before wrapping it around myself, tucking in the top corner under my armpit.

The white bath mat is soft and warm as I step out of the shower, droplets of water rolling down my ankles and pooling on the thick, worn knit. The mirror is partially fogged over, but I can still see myself looking back at me, taking in the changes: the short hair; the divot on my forehead that looks more like a strangely-placed wrinkle than a vice mark; the almost imperceptible tenseness that holds me ready to wince at a moment's notice whenever a headache might strike; the nervous waiting for it all to go to hell with a seizure; the wise gratitude that has replaced the hopeful naivete; the palpable love that surrounds me everywhere I go. I absentmindedly run my finger down the length of my scar, like I have so many times since it was put there. Thank you, God.

I lift the towel to my head, scrubbing it dry and making the scent of the conditioner wash over me. I pick up the old silk robe that lay on the floor, tying it into a bow at my hip and survey myself. Is everything perfect? No, but what in life is? I can live with headaches and the occasional strange sensation just fine. Someday I'll be able to sleep on my left again, but I've learned so much about the world and about myself that it's a small price to pay for my new lease on life.

# Thank You

Where to even start? In no particular order, thank you to everyone who helped me on this journey. You gave me the strength and courage to change my life. Thank you to all of my readers, both of this book and of the blog. Thank you to everyone who held my hand, prayed for me, sent me good luck and healing vibes - they worked! Thank you to Eve and Jill for your unending support and for keeping everyone up to date when I couldn't, even though I didn't have them shave my head. Thank you to Kendra, Coco and Greta for being the best sisters anyone could ask for. Thank you to my doctors, nurses and technicians for fixing me. Thank you to Sydney for holding my hand and comforting me as I went under. Thank you to Martha for catching my barf and to all of my aunts and uncles (Paul, I include you in that) for visiting me both in and after the hospital. Thank you to Team Erica in Minnesota, Colorado, Wisconsin and literally all over the world for always being with me through every step of the way. Thank you to John for everything you are; I love you more every day. Lastly, thank you to my parents: you are an inspiration to me for everything a parent should be. You've given me life and a new life and always stick with me.

I love you all and always will.

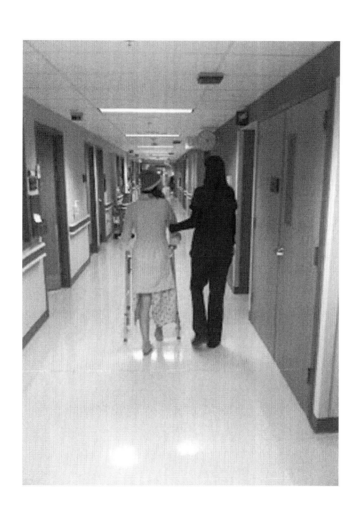

Made in the USA
Lexington, KY
24 July 2013